7882

Quality Control

METHODS IN HEMATOLOGY

Volume 4

EDITORIAL BOARD

I. Chanarin, MD, FRCPath, *Chairman*
   Northwick Park Hospital and Clinical Research Centre
   London, England

Ernest Beutler, MD
   Scripps Clinic and Research Foundation
   La Jolla, California

Elmer B. Brown, MD
   Washington University School of Medicine
   St. Louis, Missouri

Allan Jacobs, MD, FRCPath
   Welsh National School of Medicine
   Cardiff, Wales

Also in the Series

Volume 1: Iron, James D. Cook, *Guest Editor*
Volume 2: The Leukemic Cell, D. Catovsky, *Guest Editor*
Volume 3: Leucocyte Function, Martin J. Cline, *Guest Editor*

Forthcoming Volumes in the Series

Volume 5: The Hemophilias, Arthur Bloom, *Guest Editor*
Volume 6: The Thalassemias, David Weatherall, *Guest Editor*
Volume 7: Disorders of Thrombin Formation, Robert Colman, *Guest Editor*
Volume 8: The Immune Cytopenias, Robert McMillan, *Guest Editor*
Volume 9: The Cobalamins, Charles Hall, *Guest Editor*

Quality Control

EDITED BY

I. Cavill PhD, MRCPath

Senior Lecturer in Haematology,
Welsh National School of Medicine,
Cardiff, Wales

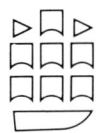

CHURCHILL LIVINGSTONE
EDINBURGH LONDON MELBOURNE AND NEW YORK 1982

CHURCHILL LIVINGSTONE
Medical Division of Longman Group Limited

Distributed in the United States of America by Churchill Livingstone Inc., 19 West 44th Street, New York, N.Y. 10036, and by associated companies, branches and representatives throughout the world.

© Longman Group Limited, 1982

All rights reserved. No part of this publication may be reproduced, stored in a retrieval system, or transmitted in any form or by any means, electronic, mechanical, photocopying, recording or otherwise, without the prior permission of the publishers (Churchill Livingstone, Robert Stevenson House, 1–3 Baxter's Place, Leith Walk, Edinburgh, EH1 3AF).

First published 1982

ISBN 0 443 02229 1

British Library Cataloguing in Publication Data
Quality control. — (Methods in hematology; 3)
  1. Blood — Examinations — Techniques
  I. Cavill, I.   II. Series
  616.07'561   RB45

Library of Congress Catalog Card Number 81-68801

Printed in Great Britain by
Butler & Tanner Ltd, Frome and London

Preface

The problem of controlling the quality of output of the modern hematology laboratory is in essence the same as that created by automation or industrialization in other spheres. The statistical foreword to this volume, Chapter 1, provides a link to the industrial origins of quality control techniques and shows that we do not need to develop these statistics but simply to learn how to apply them in the hematology laboratory. These techniques are understandably more readily applied to automated routine blood counting than to many other aspects of hematology. Nevertheless, there are other real problems in standardizing automated blood counters. The practical difficulties that may be encountered and the controls necessary are described in this volume from the point of view of the Coulter system but apply equally to other families of instruments. Automated blood counting is not the only area of hematology where there is difficulty in standardizing apparatus and methods. In many circumstances, particularly in relation to blood group serology and coagulation assays, the answer still lies in defining standard methods and standard reagents.

When estimations are carried out only occasionally, continuity between the separate batches of assays can only be maintained by strict control of methodological variation. The approach and methods described for such control could well be applied to all aspects of laboratory methods. The difficulties that are involved in assessing the efficacy of standardization procedures in the individual laboratory by means of interlaboratory trials are best illustrated in routine blood counting. In the absence of any absolute yardstick there is very great difficulty in deciding the true value of any particular parameter. Interlaboratory schemes can perform a crucial role in promoting uniformity between laboratories even if it is, theoretically, possible that they are equally wrong.

Within each laboratory and between each point at which an instrument or method is calibrated the quality of results from sample to sample must remain the same. In hematology there are two different approaches to such interlaboratory quality control. Either patients' data or the results from control samples may be analyzed. The correct methods in relation to each procedure are described by their respective protagonists. Whichever approach is used for routine blood counting can also be extended to all the other quantitative assays that the laboratory undertakes. It seems increasingly likely that in the future one or both of these approaches may be incorporated in the automated blood counter itself. At that point it will be even more important for the hematologist to understand what the machine is doing if he or she is to retain mastery over the apparatus.

Cardiff, 1982   I.C.

Contributors

T.W. Barrowcliffe, PhD
Scientist, National Institute for Biological Standards and Control, London

A.F. Bissell, PhD, FIS
Consultant and Lecturer in Applied Statistics, Abergavenny, Wales

B.S. Bull, MD
Professor and Chairman, Department of Pathology and Laboratory Medicine, Loma Linda University, California

I. Cavill, PhD, MRCPath
Senior Lecturer in Haematology, Welsh National School of Medicine, Cardiff, Wales

J.S.L. Fowler, BVM&S, MRCVS, PhD
Section for Clinical Toxicology, Safety of Medicines Department, ICI Ltd., Macclesfield, England

J.M. Gibson, ANZIMLS
Applications Manager, Coulter Electronics Ltd., Luton, England

A.M. Holburn, MB ChB, MRCPath
Director, Blood Group Reference Laboratory, London

A. Jacobs, MD, FRCP, FRCPath
Professor of Haematology, Welsh National School of Medicine, Cardiff, Wales

R.A. Korpman, MD
Assistant Professor Department of Laboratory and Pathology Medicine, Loma Linda University, California.

S.M. Lewis, BSc, MD, FRCPath
Reader in Haematology, Royal Postgraduate Medical School, London

C. Ricketts, PhD
Scientific Officer, Department of Haematology, University Hospital of Wales, Cardiff, Wales

P.G. Ward, AIBiol, AIMLS, LRSC
Scientific Officer, UK National External Quality Assessment Scheme for Haematology, Department of Haematology, Royal Postgraduate Medical School, London

Jane M. Wardle, AIMLS
Senior Medical Laboratory Scientific Officer, UK National External Quality Assessment Scheme for Haematology, Department of Haematology, Royal Postgraduate Medical School, London

Contents

1. Statistical Foreword — A.F. Bissell — 1
2. Standardization for Routine Blood Counting — J.M. Gibson — 13
3. Quality Assurance and Standardization in Blood Group Serology — A.M. Holburn — 34
4. Standardization of Coagulation Tests and Assays — T.W. Barrowcliffe — 51
5. Quality Control of Batch Assays — J.S.L. Fowler — 87
6. Standardization for Routine Blood Counting — The Role of Interlaboratory Trials — P.G. Ward J. Wardle S.M. Lewis — 102
7. Intralaboratory Quality Control using Patients' Data — B.S. Bull R.A. Korpman — 121
8. Intralaboratory Quality Control using Control Samples — C. Ricketts — 151
9. Interpretation and Significance of Laboratory Results — I. Cavill A. Jacobs — 173

Appendix: Simple statistics — 182

Index — 187

1
Statistical Foreword
A.F. Bissell

The object of this chapter is to first trace the development of quality control from its early applications in mass production to its present widespread use in industry, commerce and medicine. The second objective is to outline those statistical concepts on which quality control methods depend.

Although some early applications of statistics to industrial problems can be traced to the 19th century, the formal beginning of statistical quality control dates from the 1920s.[1] Development continued through the 1930s.[2] Military needs for large numbers of items produced to high quality standards brought a great diversity of applications and this was accelerated by the industrial recovery of the major nations after the war, although few fundamentally new methods emerged until the middle 1950s.[3,4] The success of these new techniques led to the realization that they could also be applied to other activities where maintenance of a satisfactory level of 'quality' — whether goods or services — was important.[5,6]

The development of quality control has been along two distinct lines. One of these related to a form of control in which data obtained from observation of a process was used to influence its manner of operation ('feedback'). The other line (quality assurance or quality audit) was concerned with the acceptance or rejection of batches of items based on inspection or testing of a sample. Feedback in this case is tenuous and only if there is some indirect signal, such as inability to sell his goods, might the manufacturer be induced to improve his performance. In this book we are concerned with those methods of quality control which will result in decisions about the process rather than with quality audit. The aim is to maintain the quality of the output by interacting with the process.

Why was quality control found to be necessary? In the era of craft industry each craftsman ensured that every item he produced was of good quality, at least to his own satisfaction. After the industrial revolution, and especially with the advent of high speed mass production techniques, the machine operator could exercise only a very general control by exploiting the inherent capabilities of his machine to the best advantage. Further, his role in the production of a complete product was probably small, in that he might only be producing one of many components to be assembled in the final article. The craftsman could 'fettle' components so that they matched or fitted, but such individual attention was impracticable in mass production. It was for this reason that the specification of quality requirements became a critical aspect of the complete manufacturing process. The need then was for a means of ensuring that these criteria were being observed.

CONTROL CHARTS

Early quality control methods were directed towards the production of large numbers of nominally identical items — engineering components, electric light bulbs, glass bottles, etc. Small samples, comprising from two to ten items depending on circumstances, were taken from the production line for inspection or for the measurement of some quality characteristic (freedom from defects, physical dimensions, a strength property, etc.). Provided that the sample data were compatible with the natural variation expected under satisfactory (target) conditions, no further action was required. Evidence of some significant departure outside this natural variation was deemed to justify 'action'. Such action might be minor correction of a machine setting, worn cutting tools or other components, or complete suspension of manufacture for further investigation.

A simple means of rapidly assessing the data was needed close to the manufacturing process and this is how control charts originated. The data from each sample were generally plotted on a display and lines were drawn across the chart to indicate the range of natural variation. The occurrence of plotted points outside the control lines was taken as the warning signal, whilst the absence of any violation of the lines was taken to mean that the process could continue to run uninterrupted.

FURTHER APPLICATIONS

The success of these early applications in a few major American and British companies encouraged their adaptation to other kinds of manufacturing processes. These often differed in important aspects from the mass production line. For example, chemical processes (where the product may be a liquid, slurry, powder or gas, rather than a stream of discrete items) were found to be readily susceptible to improvement by statistical control methods.[5] Similarly, products of a semi-continuous nature, such as paper, textile fabrics and wire could similarly be controlled, subject to the limitations of access for sampling.

During the last 30 years, it has been increasingly recognized that the basic philosophy of statistical quality control is relevant to almost any situation where it is necessary or desirable to monitor the output of a system in order to detect changes in its performance. The first applications in this wider context were not far removed from industrial quality control — monitoring customer complaint rates, controlling the contents of pre-packaged goods, measuring changes in productivity. More recently, statistical control methods have been extended to monitoring expenditure, error rates in clerical or card-punching operations, and even (for insurance purposes) the frequency of occurrence of defects in ships, as well as road accident rates for various classes of vehicles or drivers. Control techniques have even been used in monitoring patients' response to therapy.

LABORATORY QUALITY CONTROL

It is in connection with these wider applications beyond manufacturing industry that we find statistical quality control relevant to the laboratory in general — and to the hematological and chemical pathology laboratories in particular. Quality in laboratory tests must be related to the reliability of the results provided to the clinician. This reliability has two components which deserve immediate definition. The first is *accuracy* — the absence of systematic bias in the test method itself or on the part of the person carrying out the test. The second aspect of laboratory quality is that of *precision*. To define this term it must first be recognized that even when repeated measurements are made under apparently identical conditions the observed results will show some variation. A test method producing only small 'errors' among repeated tests is precise; one that produces widely scattered values is undesirable, in that there is doubt as to what constitutes the 'true' value of the property tested.

There may, in fact, be even more room for imprecision. Many test procedures are destructive in that individual specimens cannot be tested more than once. Repeat determinations then involve different specimens which may vary slightly from each other. This variation between specimens is then superimposed on any imprecision of the test method itself, and these two components of uncertainty are generally inseparable. Other factors may also affect the results obtained — the manner in which samples are taken from the bulk that they are supposed to represent; the effects of extraneous conditions at the time of sampling or during transit from sampling point to laboratory. This may prejudice both accuracy and precision, and hence the validity of the information that the laboratory data provides to the clinician.

As in industry, the pressures of routine testing to tight time schedules and the development of automatic devices have brought a change from the situation where a laboratory worker could (like a craftsman) concentrate on one measurement until fully satisfied of its validity. The function of quality control in hematology is the establishment and maintenance of an acceptable level of accuracy and precision in the data provided by the laboratory, so that they may form a sound basis for clinical decisions.

MEASUREMENT AND COUNTING

At this point, it is appropriate to consider some of the statistical background to quality control techniques. This begins with the twin problems of accuracy and precision. An accurate method is one which will generally give a result which is close to the true value of the parameter. On the other hand, a precise method is one that yields closely similar values under repeated testing of the same or similar specimens. It is thus possible for a method to be accurate but imprecise, or precise but inaccurate. In fact, accuracy is largely concerned with the requirement that test results should be of the right magnitude, whilst precision is concerned with the smallness of variations between repeated determinations. In other words, accuracy is associated with average level, and precision with dispersion.

Before defining measures of average and dispersion, it must be noted that two fundamentally different types of numerical data occur in laboratory testing. The first is obtained from observations made on a continuous scale of measurement. Familiar examples of measurement are determinations of length, mass, temperature, chemical composition, etc., where (apart from limitations of equipment) the observations may take any value along a continuous scale. The other type of data is obtained by counting some kind of event or attribute. These are particularly common in hematology. Observations of blood cell concentrations, radioactive particle counts, etc. all depend on counting the number of occurrences of some phenomenon, and must necessarily yield integer values. This distinction between measurement and counting has important statistical implications but the boundary between the two types becomes blurred where the integer steps in counted data are small relative to the total number of observations. As a result, large counts may be treated in the same way as measurements on a continuous scale.

LOCATION AND DISPERSION

The quantification of accuracy and precision require a measure of location and of dispersion respectively. As far as the question of location is concerned, the *arithmetic mean* (commonly called 'the average') is the most widely used and best understood measure. Its origins are lost in antiquity, but it is based on the idea of pooling all the numerical values and sharing the total equally among all the items. If a set of n observations is denoted by the symbols X_1, X_2, X_3, etc. up to X_n, the general observation may be symbolized as X_i. The arithmetic mean is then represented by:

$$\bar{X} = \frac{1}{n} \sum_{i=1}^{i=n} X_i$$

where the Σ sign is an instruction to add all the X-values whose subscripts appear in the range 1 to n. This notation may a first appear to be an unnecessary complication, but it will prove useful at later stages both in this and later chapters.

One great advantage of the arithmetic mean is that it makes use of all the observations in a set of data. This is less true of some other measures of location such as the median (the central value when the observations are ordered in magnitude) or the mode (the most frequently occurring value or the region on the scale of measurement where values cluster most thickly). However, the median is a useful alternative to the mean in some circumstances.

One intuitive measure of dispersion is the range of a set of values, that is, the difference between the largest and smallest value. Although attractively simple, it has two disadvantages. The first is that it is susceptible to the influence of individual wild values. In addition it does not lend itself to the comparison of dispersions among groups having differing numbers of observations. *The variance*, on the other hand, provides a measure of variation that (like the mean) depends on all the values. Using the previous notation it is given by:

$$\text{Var} = \frac{1}{n-1} \sum_{i=1}^{i=n} (X - \bar{X})^2$$

i.e. approximately the mean of the squared deviations of the X-values from their arithmetic mean. The divisor n-1, rather than n, is generally adopted when estimating dispersion from a sample, and an account of the justification for this will be found in many statistical texts. Unfortunately, the variance is not readily interpretable in terms of the original scale of measurement of X, but its square root returns it to the original dimensions of measurement. This is known as the *standard deviation* and is defined thus:

$$\text{SD} = \sqrt{\frac{1}{n-1} \Sigma (X - \bar{X})^2}$$

SAMPLES AND POPULATIONS

In most collections of numerical data, the observations comprise only a portion of all the possible values of the variable of interest. In particular, when considering quality control applications, many items may be manufactured but only a few will be measured or tested. Similarly in the laboratory, checks on accuracy and precision can only be made occasionally and not alongside every analytical determination of a routine test. The set of all possible values (which may often be intangible or hypothetical) is known as the *population*. The extent to which statistics (such as $\bar{X}$ and SD) represent the corresponding true parameters of the population (say μ and σ) depends on the manner of selection of samples, on the size of the sample, and on the correct choice of sample statistic. Whenever variation occurs, it is inevitable that different samples will provide varying estimates of the corresponding population parameters. Under ideal conditions of random sampling from a single stable population the variation among sample estimates of the arithmetic mean is represented by the *standard error* of the sample mean. This is analagous to the standard deviation of individual values. For samples of size n, the standard error is given by:

$$\text{standard error of } \bar{X} = \frac{\text{SD}}{\sqrt{n}}$$

In hematological practice the relation between population and sample may be illustrated in terms of the use of one (or a few) blood samples to provide an estimate of blood 'quality' for the whole individual. In the same way we may use a small number of measurements of a control sample to provide an indication of overall performance of the counter over a given time period. Both estimates of the truth will be subject to sampling variation, which may be estimated from the standard deviation, and the means of repeated samples will vary with a variation described by the standard error.

6 QUALITY CONTROL

DISTRIBUTION AND PROBABILITY

When numerical data are obtained the values show variations which are *distributed* along the appropriate scale of measurement. Bar charts and histograms are familiar methods of illustrating these distributions of empirical observations. It has been found that some basic patterns of distribution occur frequently, and that they can be represented by mathematical formulae which greatly facilitate the handling of data in statistical analysis. In order to compare distributions in groups comprising varying numbers of observations it is preferable to consider the relative, rather than absolute, frequencies of occurrence of the various values. The relative frequencies with which particular values occur are then analogous to the probabilities of their appearance under random sampling from the parent population. Probability is measured on the scale zero (impossibility) to one (certainty) and we thus have, for a population of values or for a theoretical distribution,

$$\text{Probability of occurrence of a particular value, x} = \frac{\text{frequency of occurrence of x}}{\text{sum of frequencies of all possible values}}$$

As in the case of estimating parameters (e.g. μ, σ) from sample values ($\bar{x}$, s), probabilities also need to be estimated, directly or indirectly, from sample data. Theoretical distributions often provide the means of relating sample statistics to relative frequencies or probabilities. Biological data may involve three such distributions, two concerned with counted data and one with measurements.

1. *The Binomial distribution* is concerned with the counts of binary events where each observation is a record of whether some attribute is present or absent. An everyday example is tossing a coin, where it may fall heads or not (if not, it is presumed to fall tails); similarly in inspecting manufactured items, each is or is not defective, there are no half-measures or gradations.

When a random sample of n such observations is obtained from a population, system or process in which a proportion, p, of items have the attribute of interest, then the probability distribution of the number of items, r, in the sample having that attribute can be expressed in terms of the parameters n and p. It is also useful to introduce the auxiliary parameter $q = 1 - p$ to simplify the expression, which is:

$$\Pr(r) = \frac{n!}{r!(n-r)!} \cdot p^r \cdot q^{n-r}$$

The mean number of occurrences per group of n observations is np, and the variance npq. The valid application of the Binomial model hinges on the assumptions that occurrences of the attribute are mutually independent (for example, that one occurrence neither prompts nor inhibits others), and that the probability of individual occurrences is homogeneous over the whole population or system.

2. *The Poisson distribution* is also concerned with counted events, but of a different type. Here the events are not binary, but comprise the occurrence of some phenomenon in a continuum. Examples are the rate of accidents in equal

intervals of time, or the concentration of suspended particles in a fluid medium. It assumes that the overall rate of occurrence, say λ events per unit of observation on the continuum, is stable, but that the events occur at random points in the continuum. The probability of occurrence of exactly r events in a unit of observation is then:

$$\Pr(r) = e^{-\lambda} \cdot \frac{\lambda r}{r!}.$$

The mean and variance of the distribution are both λ so that the standard deviation is simply $\sqrt{\lambda}$. It may be noted that the Poisson model also provides a useful approximation in Binomial distributions whose proportion parameter, p, is small (say less than 0.1). This is achieved by taking λ = np (equating the mean of the Poisson distribution to that of the Binomial).

3. The most useful of the statistical models for variables measured on a continuous scale is *the Normal (or Gaussian) distribution*. It arises from the 'theory of errors' in which many small, independent and additive sources of error are supposed to contribute to an overall departure from a hypothetical true value. The resulting distribution of total error is characterised by the standard deviation, σ, and the distribution is symmetrical about the true value, μ. The shape of the curve representing the Normal distribution (its 'density function') is given by

$$f(x) = \frac{1}{\sigma\sqrt{2\pi}} \exp\left[-\frac{1}{2}\left(\frac{x-\mu}{\sigma}\right)^2\right]$$

and the integral of this expression with respect to x gives the distribution function. The difference between the values of the integral for any pair of x values (x_1, x_2) yields the probability of occurrence of an observation in the range x_1 to x_2. No general expression for this integral exists, but the distribution with λ = 0, σ = 1 is tabulated in most statistical text books. Any other Normal distribution is reduced to this standard form by writing

$$u = \frac{x - \mu}{\sigma}$$

where μ and σ are the mean and standard deviation of the distribution from which x is an observation. The Normal distribution is symmetrical, with a central mode (Fig. 1.1). Approximately two-thirds (more exactly 68.27 per cent)

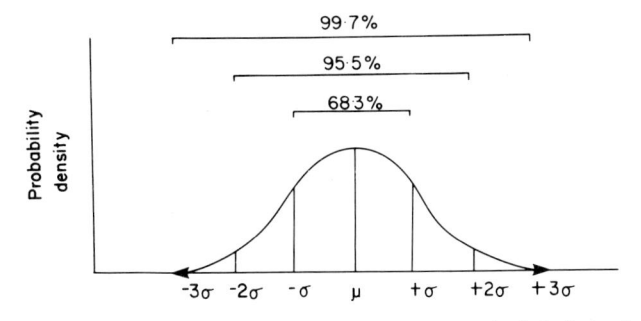

Fig. 1.1 The Normal distribution about the mean (μ) which its standard deviation (σ).

of the distribution is covered by the range $\mu-\sigma$ to $\mu + \sigma$, about 95.5 per cent by the range $\mu-2\sigma$, and most (99.7%) by the range $\mu-3\sigma$ to $\mu + 3\sigma$.

The range of application of the Normal distribution is greatly extended by the use of transformations of asymetrically distributed variables. The most common transform involves taking the logarithm of variables whose distributions have long upper tails but short lower tails or the square root for the opposite distribution. The main importance of the Normal distribution arises from the Central Limit Theorem. This derives from the observation that when the variable of interest is itself the average of several (or many) contributing measurements then the distribution of such sample averages is more nearly Normal than that of the individual contributions. Further, the sample averages are less widely dispersed than the individual observations so that for samples of size n the distribution of x (the mean of n observations) tends towards a Normal distribution with μ and standard error $\sigma/\sqrt{n}$ (the parameters μ, σ, refer to the distribution of individual values). Although the standard error is used in an identical manner to the standard deviation, the two terms are used to avoid confusion between variation of sample statistics and variation among individual values.

Examples of all three of these distribution models arise in hematological applications. Counting one group of blood cells from amongst a larger number of other cells provides an application of the Binomial distribution. The Poisson distribution describes the variation of all counts of radioactivity and also the frequency of occurrence of different cell types, as in the white cell differential. When the number of cells counted becomes large, as in the Coulter white and red cell count, then they may be treated as observations on a continuous scale and the Normal distribution or a transformation may provide a suitable model.

QUALITY CONTROL

The essential feature of statistical quality control techniques is that a target distribution is specified. This target distribution, which may be Binomial, Poisson, Normal or even of some other form, describes the expected pattern of variation in a relevant sample statistic. The object is then to detect any important change from the target conditions. Such changes will usually involve one of the following although other possibilities do exist.

1. An increase in the value of p when the Binomial model is used to represent a target distribution; for example the numbers of defective items found in samples of size n.
2. A change in the value of λ when the Poisson model represents the distribution; e.g. the numbers of faults in samples of cloth, wire, etc.
3. A change in the mean value (μ) or the variability as measured by (σ) in a Normal distribution representing values of a critical variable.

Numerous statistical procedures are used in quality control, but they all fall under three main headings:
1. Stochastic (i.e. based on interacting probabilities) models of the behaviour of a series with time.
2. Control charts.
3. Cumulative sum (Cusum) procedures.

Stochastic methods require an extensive analysis of the past behaviour of a series of data. From this a model is constructed which from past experience is able to predict forthcoming observations. If the predicted values deviate from those observed in practice this indicates a departure from target conditions and a correction is prescribed.

The second and third groups of techniques are often (though not always) implemented graphically and the resulting charts provide a useful, economical summary of the data. The Cusum chart, in particular, can yield powerful diagnostic clues to anomalies in whatever process is being monitored and this point will be developed later. First the simple control chart. The data may be compromised of counts of defective items or faults, or may be measured characteristics of sampled items. These counts or measurements (or sample statistics obtained from them) are plotted in time sequence on a chart. Control limits, often termed 'action lines', are drawn on the chart indicating the range within which the observations should lie under satisfactory conditions. The occurrence of a sample value outside a control limit is regarded as a signal that the process characteristics have changed and that some action (correction, adjustment, maintenance, investigation) is required. The positioning of the limits is important, as two kinds of risk are associated with any control procedure based on sampling viz:

1. If the limits are set too close to the target value, then the natural variation in the process may yield a proportion of sample statistics violating the limits even when the process is 'in control'. Any action taken on such signals will then result in false alarms (i.e. 'false positives').
2. If the limits are set too far from the target, then important departures from satisfactory conditions may fail to yield signals, and the appropriate action may be delayed (in industry, for example, until customer complaint or production difficulties draw attention to the situation).

Commonly adopted values for control limits are those points on the target distribution which would only be reached by about 1 in 1000 samples when the process is in control (for a Normal distribution of sample means, this will correspond to about $3\sigma/\sqrt{n}$ on either side of the target, where the standard error of sample means is $\sigma/\sqrt{n}$.) (Fig. 1.2).

Secondary limits, known as 'warning lines', are often incorporated on control charts. They are generally located at the 1 in 40 points of the target distribution. For sample means this wil be at $2\sigma/\sqrt{n}$ on either side of the target. Be-

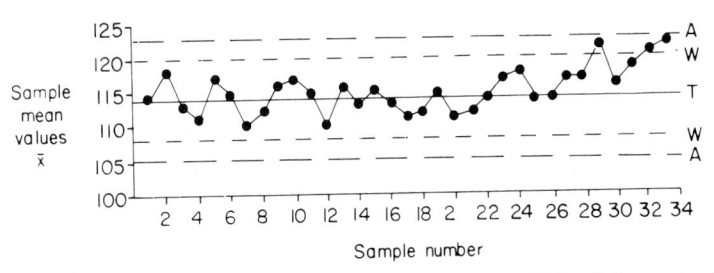

Fig. 1.2 A control chart for sample means where the target value = 114 and the standard error of each mean = 3.0. Warning lines (W) and action lines (A).

cause any action taken on isolated violations of the warning lines might produce a number of false alarm this method is often refined so that *two* successive violations of warning lines are needed to yield a signal. In this case a single crossing of the line may be regarded as an indication that the next sample should be taken earlier than usual to either confirm the out-of-control alert or to reassure the operator that the first violation was only a chance occurrence. By using limits of this kind the risk of false alarms may be controlled at one in several hundred samples.

The power of a quality control procedure to detect changes of any given magnitude depends on the sample size adopted. Because the standard error of a statistic decreases with increasing sample size, large samples offer greater response for any given change in the behaviour of a process. This aspect of QC methods has generally received scant attention. Many users have adopted a rule-of-thumb sample size of four or five almost irrespective of the sensitivity (or insensitivity) of the sample statistic to changes of a critical magnitude. The average run length before there is a significant indication of change for any particular procedure provides a measure of its rate of response to various amounts of shift from target. By inspecting such data and by plotting it in relation to sample sizes or sampling frequencies the resulting curve can be used to find an optimum sample size and frequency combination.

The control chart has the great virtue of simplicity, but is somewhat inefficient in that decisions are generally based on only the most recent one or two data values. Where detection of small but sustained changes in average level is important the Cusum type of procedure has major advantages. It is particularly applicable, for example, in the presymptomatic indication of a trend in a patient's test results or in the detection of changes in machine performance before they reach a clinically significant level. Quite apart from its efficiency in detecting changes, the Cusum chart permits the estimation of the points at which such changes occur. This in turn allows the calculation of local average values, for example, before and after calibration or over a particular reporting period. The chart also draws attention to the often overlooked fact that the point at which a change is perceived, and hence at which a decision is taken, does not usually correspond to the origin of any such change. Several samples may be taken after a deviation before the quality control procedure signals the true situation. Extrapolation back along the Cusum plot can enable the point at which the deviation occurred to be more clearly defined.

The Cusum method requires the formulation of a target value, T. This will, in most applications, be a constant, but the procedures are even adaptable to situations where the target may depend (for example) on ambient conditions, current calibration factors or some other value which may change from one constant to another. Whatever the appropriate target, its value is simply subtracted from each successive value of the sample statistic. The resulting deviations, x-T, are algebraically added (i.e. cumulatively summed) to yield the Cusum, $\Sigma(x-T)$. The current value of the Cusum is plotted (as ordinate) against the sample number or time of sampling (as abscissa). If the process is operating at or close to its Target the Cusum path progresses roughly parallel to the sample number axis. If an upward shift in average level occurs, the predominantly positive (x-T) values will produce a steadily increasing Cusum, $\Sigma(x-T)$, and the Cusum plot will slope upwards. Conversely, a downward shift in average gives a downward Cusum slope. Thus a change in average level of the plotted variable appears as a change of *slope* in the Cusum chart. This is the source of its great sensitivity but it may also have hindered its adoption by those who associate average level with chart ordinates, as in simple Control charts. As an example of the increase in sensitivity which this technique brings to analysis the data presented in Figure 1.2 is displayed as a Cusum chart in Figure 1.4.

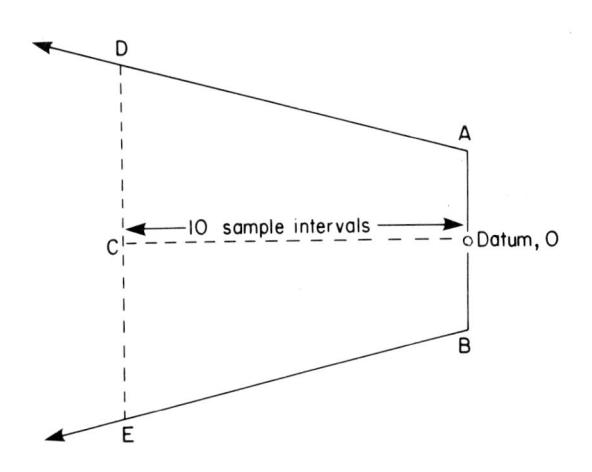

Fig. 1.3 Construction of a mask for assessing the Cusum chart.
OA = OB = 5 standard errors
CD = CE = 10 standard errors
The mask may be extended beyond D and E as required. Datum 0, is placed over the latest cusum point with OC parallel to the x-axis.

The Cusum technique is just a simple but effective method of magnifying consistent change. It works, in effect, by stripping away the largely uninteresting but predominant 'background' bulk of a variable, leaving only the sensitive portion to stand out on its own. The technique can be applied to any set of sequential data and is completely independent of the nature of the distribution of that data. If it is used in a straightforward chart then assessment of any change in slope by eye alone must be subjective. In order to remove this subjectivity it is necessary to use an explicit and objective set of rules for assessment. These decision rules will, in contrast to the Cusum itself, depend upon the nature of the distribution of the data. One means of implementing a decision rule is to construct a mask which can be placed on the chart at the most recently plotted point. For a normally distributed variable a relatively simple mask can be used. The chart scale itself is important and the scales and form of mask shown in Figure 1.3 are one of the most widely used. Taking one sample interval on the horizontal axis as the unit of measurement on the vertical scale then the Cusum is marked off in multiples of approximately two standard errors per unit distance. The half-height and slope of the mask (5 standard errors, and 0.5 standard errors per sample interval respectively) may then be con-

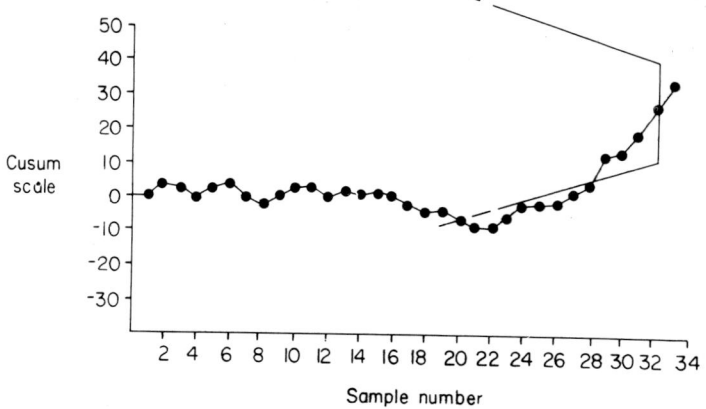

Fig. 1.4 Cusum chart of the data presented in Fig. 1.2. The mask indicates that there was a significant deviation from the Target value (114) at the 20th sample.

structed directly from the Cusum ordinate scale. It is not necessary to apply this scale convention rigorously and slight modifications for the sake of a convenient scaling factor are permissible. If the Cusum path crosses the limits of the mask (as shown in Fig. 1.4) a change in the process mean is indicated.

CONCLUDING REMARKS

This chapter provides only a brief account both of the history and the statistical basis of quality control procedures. The extension of such techniques to the clinical laboratory are part of the natural progression which has brought both science and automation into patient investigations. Detailed statistical methodologies are now available, some as British Standards Institution publications[7,8] and it is to these that the inquiring reader is directed for further exploration of this field.

REFERENCES

1. Shewhart, W A 1931 Economic control of quality of manufactured products. van Nostrand, New York
2. Pearson E S 1935 The application of statistical methods to industrial standardization and quality control. British Standard 600. British Standards Institution, London
3. Page E S 1955 Control charts with warning lines. Biometrika 42–43: 248
4. Barnard, G A 1959 Control charts and stochastic processes. Journal of the Royal Statistical Society, Series B 21: 239–271
5. Woodward R H Goldsmith P L 1964 Cumulative sum techniques. ICI monograph No. 3. Oliver and Boyd, Edinburgh
6. Bissell A F 1969 Cusum techniques for quality control. Applied Statistics 18: 1–30
7. British Standard 2564, 1955 Control chart technique when manufacturing to a specification. British Standards Institution, London
8. British Standard 5703, 1980 Data analysis and quality control using cusum techniques, Parts I and II. British Standards Institution, London

2
Standardization for Routine Blood Counting
J. M. Gibson

The only true standard in hematology is a cyanmethemoglobin solution made by the Rijks Institute at Bilthoven, Netherlands in accordance with the recommendations of the International Committee for Standards in Hematology (ICSH). The method for assaying such a primary standard is based on the extinction coefficient of a pure cyanmethemoglobin solution. This technique cannot be used on a routine basis because of the need for a pure cyanmethemoglobin solution and the high accuracy of spectrophotometry required. The world of cell counting and sizing is very poorly supplied with standards, there being no materials available as yet for calibration (primary standardization). Reference techniques do exist, however, and these have given rise to secondary standards. These are stabilized bloods usually in an embalming fluid to give a working life of a month or two. Such materials are assigned assay values from instrumentation calibrated by reference techniques. They should only be used as reference controls for such instrumentation, and not as calibrators. However, because of the reliability of many of these control preparations and because of pressures of work within some laboratories, they are often used as calibrators. In most cases this will not give rise to any problems but this is fortuitous. It must be understood that these stabilized controls have very distinct properties and may not behave in anything like the same manner as fresh blood.

The aim of this chapter is not to describe how to set up and operate equipment or how to carry out basic methods. These are already covered by operating manuals and other volumes. Rather the intention is to describe how to calibrate such equipment or methods while at the same time drawing attention to factors which may affect this and the subsequent quality of the blood counts. The problems, and their solutions, that arise in calibration often apply equally to routine operation of the blood counter.

HEMOGLOBIN

The recommended technique for the measurement of the hemoglobin concentration in whole blood is based on a fresh solution of detergent modified Drabkin's reagent[1]:

Potassium ferricyanide $K_3Fe(CN)_6$	0.200 g
Potassium cyanide KCN	0.050 g

	Potassium dihydrogen orthophosphate anhydrous KH$_2$PO$_4$	0.140 g
either	Sterox S.E.	0.5 ml
or	Nonidet P.40 or Triton X-100	1.0 ml
	distilled water to	1000 ml

This solution should have a pH of 7.0 to 7.4, be clear and pale yellow in color. When measured in a photometer at 540 nm against a water blank, the reading should be zero. For use, 1 ml of fresh blood should be diluted to 250 ml with Drabkins reagent (1:250) and allowed to react for 3 minutes (see Note 1, p. 15). During this time the cells will be lysed and their hemoglobin converted to cyanmethemoglobin. The absorbance of this solution should be read on a photometer at 540 nm.

Calibration of the photometer must be carried out using the ICSH hemoglobincyanide (cyanmethemoglobin) solution of 58.0 mg/dl ± 0.1 mg/dl (Note 2, p. 15). This solution, if stored at 0 to 4°C, should be warmed to room temperature to prevent condensation on the cuvette. Alternative standards are commercially available which have been related to the ICSH standard and may be used (see Note 3, p. 15). Do not expose the materials to any bright lights (see Note 4, p. 15). The standards should be blanked against distilled water or Drabkins reagent in matched cuvettes and the absorbance at 540 nm recorded (see Note 5, p. 15). The appropriate hemoglobin concentration for the reference solution should be calculated as $\frac{58}{1000} \times 250 = 14.5$ g/dl. Accurate dilutions (e.g. 1:2, 1:3, 1:4) of this cyanmethemoglobin solution in Drabkins reagent should be made in Drabkins solution and their absorbance measured. Beer's Law is obeyed for cyanmethemoglobin solutions at this concentration and a plot on linear paper of absorbance units on the ordinate (y axis) against hemoglobin concentration on the abscissa (x axis) should give a straight line which passes through the origin. The concentration of an unknown solution of hemoglobin can be read from this curve. The possibility that interfering substances may be present should be borne in mind (see Note 8, p. 16).

A photometer giving a direct reading of hemoglobin concentration, e.g. Coulter® hemoglobinometer, may have preset dilution factors e.g. 1:501 and 1:251. This type of instrument generally uses a flow-through cuvette and measures a blank automatically after each cycle. The blank solution must, therefore, have zero absorbance. Any particulate material or detectable color would falsely elevate the blank absorbances and thereby depress the apparent hemoglobin concentration. Air bubbles in the flow and pump lines will have the same effect. The instrument should be calibrated by adjusting the readout (see manufacturer's instruction manual) to give the correct reading for the reference solution at the appropriate dilution. Dilutions of the standard should be measured and the observed hemoglobin concentration plotted against the calculated value. This should give a straight line with zero intercept. Never assume that there is linearity and a zero intercept: verify it.

Commercial Drabkins reagent solutions should be freshly prepared before use (see Note 6, p. 16). Other commercial alternatives to Drabkins reagent, for example those produced by Coulter Electronics, Isoton® II (a buffered, filtered diluent) and Zapoglobin® (a red cell stromatolyzing solution which leaves white cells for counting and converts the released hemoglobin to the cyanmethemoglobin form) should only be used as recommended by the manufacturers.

If an automatic diluter is used (see Note 7, p. 16) it must be calibrated by comparison with accurate manual dilutions of cyamethamoglobin as above. It cannot be assumed that the diluter is correct. The calibration of multiparameter automated cell counters (see Note 8, p. 16) is an extension of the calibration of diluters and automated photometers.

Note 1

The conversion time for hemoglobin to cyanmethemoglobin is three minutes for fresh blood in detergent modified Drabkins solution. During this time stromatolysis proceeds to ensure a clear, particle-free solution of cyanmethemoglobin. This should be stable for at least one hour if protected from strong light. Preserved whole blood preparations may take up to 10 minutes for full conversion.

Note 2

Dilution inaccuracies are often the greatest source of error in deriving the true hemoglobin content of a blood sample. Scaling the dilution down from 1 ml blood made up to 250 ml of lytic diluent introduces further errors in accuracy and precision. Altering the dilution ratio should in theory be acceptable, but the spectrophotometer may well be affected by the varying degree of stroma present (see Note 5). It is important, however, to know the true dilution that is being used. This is especially true if a variant method and lytic agent are being used. For example if 40 μl blood is diluted in 20 ml Isoton® II and lysed by the addition of 0.2 ml Zapoglobin® then the true dilution is 40 in 20 240, i.e. 1:505. If a 1:500 ratio were used to calculate the results then these would all be 1.2 per cent too low: an unnecessary additional error. The use of liquid K_3EDTA anticoagulant may add a further 1 per cent to the dilution and this should be included in the calculation.

Note 3

Commercial standards which purport to conform to the ICSH specification have been found to differ by 3 or 4 mg at the 58 mg level. Cross-checking standards from two manufacturers is recommended.

Note 4

Cyanmethemoglobin solutions are photolabile. In filter photometers where the filter is in front of the photocell, instead of in front of the sample, any prolongation of exposure to the bright light of the lamp may bleach such solutions. The absorbance should be read without delay.

Note 5

The photometer or spectrophotometer should be used with care. It is theoretically possible to use the millimolar extinction coefficient of cyamethemoglobin and the absorbance at 540 nm to calculate its concentration. However, this can only be done on a pure solution having $A_{540}:A_{504}$ ratio of 1.59 or better, with a light path of 1.000 cm ± 0.005 cm and a carefully calibrated wavelength and absorbance scale (e.g. US National Bureau of Standards filter set 930B) which will read to 0.002 absorbance units. Such systems may require environmental control cabinets. Filtering or centrifuging the hemoglobin solution is necessary to achieve the 1.59 ratio and to ensure that the absorbance at 750 nm is less than 0.002 absorbance units. This is obviously not a practicable technique for routine measurement and there is some evidence that hemoglobin can be absorbed onto the filter material.

Individual optical design will make one type of spectrophotometer more, or less, sensitive to scattered light from the white cells or red cell stroma. A simple filter photometer often gives the best reading with little error due to light scatter. The more sophisticated the instrument the more problems are likely to occur.

Note 6

The shelf life of some reagents must be considered. Open vials will lose cyanide at a rate dependent on temperature. This loss will lead to an inability to form the cyanmet complex. Drabkins reagent is also sensitive to light. No reagent should be used beyond the expiry date. Commercial lytic reagent such as Zapoglobin® should be stored carefully; if it is refrigerated, a precipitate will form; if it is exposed to bright sunlight, needle shaped crystals will precipitate and brown discoloration will occur.

Note 7

Automatic instrumentation should be carefully checked. Diluters must deliver the full volume with no air bubbles. Photometers must be set to the correct dilution and automatic cuvettes should operate freely. Fibrin clots or glass splinters from calibrator ampoules can cause faulty drainage; air leaks on rinse lines can also cause problems. Reproducibility should be checked using a large homogeneous volume of freshly prepared cyanmethemoglobin. Calibration and linearity should also be checked periodically. Instruments should not be operated with the photocell housing removed as errors may be caused by extraneous light. Home-made lytic agents such as hexadecyl-dimethyl-ammonium bromide in saline will give methemoglobin only and cannot be used in a reference method.

Note 8

Automated cell counters which take whole blood samples must be calibrated indirectly. That is, the hemoglobin concentration of 10 normal samples must first be determined independently by reference methods. This number is chosen in order to give an adequate estimate of the true mean of the samples; 20 normal samples would give a better estimate and would be preferable if time and circumstances permitted. The mean value thus ascribed to the samples should then be used to standardize the automated counter. There is a choice as to whether fresh or preserved samples are used for this purpose.

If fresh whole blood samples are used there are a number of potential problems which must be borne in mind. In general, these mainly centre on nonspecific changes in absorbance which are not related to hemoglobin concentration. Cold agglutinates will take more time to lyse and disperse;[2] hyperlipemia[3,4,5] and macroglobulinemia[6] will increase background turbidity, and the presence of large numbers of white cells (white cell counts greater than $30 \times 10^9/l$) or fatty droplets will lead to light scattering. Some heparins will interact with lytic agents such as Zapoglobin® or Coulter® Lyse S. This will cause increased turbidity which at the recommended level of 10 to 20 units heparin per ml of blood may increase the apparent hemoglobin concentration by 3 to 5 per cent, an unacceptable error. Beware of heparin coated capillary tubes for fingerprick samples. EDTA (Na_2 or K_2) are the anticoagulants of choice. The use of 10 fresh blood samples from normal individuals should minimize these problems and the apparatus should be set equal to their mean hemoglobin concentration.

The difficulties associated with choosing 10 fresh whole blood samples to calibrate automated instruments can be obviated by using stable preserved preparations. However, the red cells in such preparations as Coulter® 4C or those described in Chapters 6 and 8 show increased resistance to cell lysis. It is therefore essential to use Nonidet or Sterox detergents to completely solubilize the red cell stroma in order to obtain an accurate measure of their hemoglobin content. Incomplete stromatolysis, which in turn produced turbidity, is the most likely explanation for discrepancies reported in the hemoglobin concentration measured in commercial preparations by the ICSH recommended method.[7,8] Adequate methodology may thus allow stabilized red cell preparations to be used for calibration purposes. In the Coulter S, at least, there is no evidence that the slower rate of conversion of hemoglobin to cyanmethemoglobin in these materials has any affect on the calibration of the instrument (see Note 9).

Whether fresh or preserved bloods are used to provide a standard to which the automated blood counter should be calibrated, it is obviously important to ensure that the instrument is functioning correctly. Dirty, protein-coated baths will cause loss of sensitivity and sunlight reflected onto the photocell will cause significant errors and loss of accuracy. In the Coulter S, bubbling should be carefully adjusted so that two large bubbles rise quickly through the baths. Too high a vacuum on prediluted samples may create persistent micro-bubbles which will increase the apparent hemoglobin concentration.

Note 9

It has been shown that there is a difference in the rate at which hemoglobin is converted to cyanmethemoglobin between Coulter 4C and fresh blood (Fig. 2.1).[9] The results suggested that 4C conversion might be incomplete in the Coulter S. However this study was carried out using a narrow band-pass spectrophotometer which distinguished between met- and cyanmethemoglobin.

Direct monitoring of the photometer output from the Coulter S Junior showed that a stable reading for 4C was obtained after six seconds (Fig. 2.2). This is eight seconds before the time at which the photometer output is used by this instrument to derive the hemoglobin concentration. The explanation for this appears to lie in the optical system of the Coulter S family. This uses a

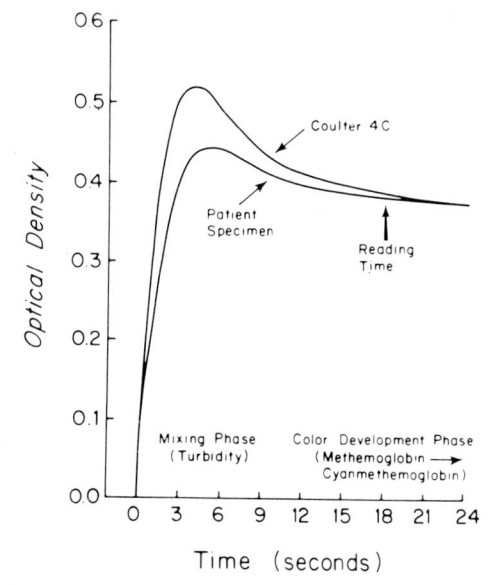

Fig. 2.1 Rates of color development of a preserved and a fresh blood sample in Drabkin's solution. Optical density was measured at 540 mm. (From Koepke 1977, with permission.)

simple filter with a peak at 525 nm and a band-pass of ± 60 nm. Readings with this system give the same absorbances for all forms of hemoglobin. Thus although both forms of hemoglobin may still be present they will give equal

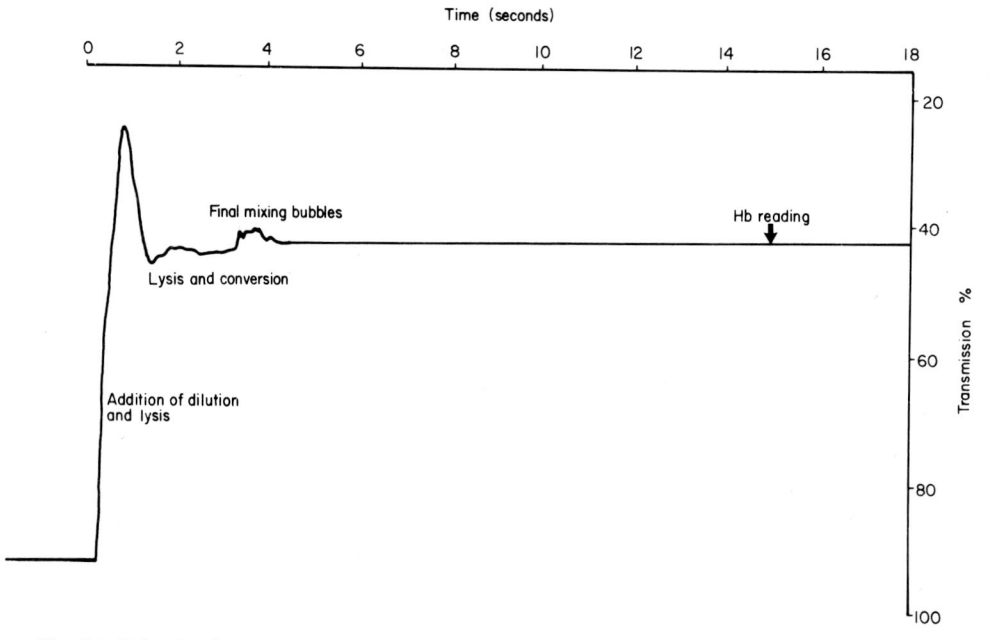

Fig. 2.2 Color development of a preserved blood sample (Coulter 4C) in Isoton® measured in a Coulter S Junior.

absorbance and hence contribute equally to the calculated hemoglobin concentration.

The stability of the photometer output during cyanmethemoglobin conversion in the Model S using Isoton® II and Lyse S can be confirmed by monitoring the 'amp output' socket on the instrument. This will give a picture similar to that shown in Figure 2.2. The voltage is stable from the time the last bubbles rise clear until many minutes later. There are some 20 seconds before this mixture is read on the Coulter S. Stability of the electronics can be shown by injecting a sample of cyanmethemoglobin solution into the WBC aperture bath during an automatic cycle instead of using the lysing (Cl) chamber output solution, which should be allowed to go to waste. The hemoglobinometer will read this relative to the blank solution of Isoton. The nominal 1:250 dilution used in the Coulter S cannot be taken as accurate for calibration purposes. Hemoglobin estimation on this instrument is thus measured by a comparator. The relationship between the photometer output and the calculated hemoglobin concentration is determined only by the calibration procedure.

CELL COUNTING AND SIZING

Electronic digital cell counting has transformed the precision of routine blood counts. Whereas coefficients of variation in the order of 12 per cent were the best that could be achieved for manual red or white cell counts, these can be reliably reduced to better than 3 per cent on automated instruments.[10] These methods are generally based on non-optical one-by-one counting of the displacement of electrolyte. A manometer or regulated vacuum source ensures that a specified amount of cellular material, suspended in an electrolyte which does not affect the cells, flows through a fine aperture of specified dimensions. A current passes between two electrodes, one on either side of the aperture which is supported in an insulating holder. As a cell passes through the aperture it displaces electrolyte. This changes the impedance between the two electrodes which in turn produces a voltage or current pulse whose magnitude is proportional to the volume of the cell.

There are a number of factors which may affect the accuracy of all pulse counting and analyzing instruments:

A. Electronic noise from other equipment can interfere and can increase the apparent count. Background counts should be consistent and negligible (see Note 4, p. 23). Noise should be absent from the oscilloscope monitor which is usually a part of these counters.

B. Air leaks in the manometer or vacuum sample system may give rise to considerable count variations and can be seen as a stream of fine bubbles within the glassware. There should be no air bubbles adhering to the platinum electrodes or glass surfaces.

C. If a manometer is used it must be clear and free of moisture and show no separation of the mercury nor trails of mercury in the horizontal metering section.

D. The aperture tube must be absolutely clean. Any protein build-up in the aperture will give an apparent increase in volume of the particles for a given size threshold. It will also allow previously excluded material below the threshold volume to appear in the 'counting window'. Thus for a fixed threshold manometer counting system the count and MCV will increase disproportionately. For the constant vacuum instruments, like the Coulter® model S, the fixed four-second count will sample less and give a lower count while the 'MCV' will appear to increase.

To prevent this occurrence, aperture tubes should be cleaned at least once a week (preferably daily, or every 500 samples). They should be removed from the instrument and soaked for 15 minutes in bleach solution then rinsed in clean electrolyte.

The bleach used should be laboratory grade sodium hypochlorite diluted 1:4 in electrolyte or distilled water (to prevent precipitates). Sodium hypochlorite is usually available as an 8 per cent stock and should be diluted down to 2 per cent available chlorine. DO NOT USE HOUSEHOLD BLEACHES containing detergents. The cationic detergents present will interact with lysing agents causing deposits on glassware. Cationic detergents act by coating glassware, making them impossible to wash clean, and will make it impossible to measure cell size. They may also cause protein to build up more rapidly around the aperture. Should these or other types of detergents (e.g. Decon, RBS, etc), have been used then the glassware should be soaked for 15 minutes in a nonionic detergent, e.g. 10 per cent Teepol L in distilled water.

Where the aperture tubes cannot be removed (e.g. Coulter S) the same preventative maintenance schedule should be followed. The aperture baths should be filled with diluted hypochlorite and then the count button pressed until the bleach enters the isolating chamber. It should be left for 15 minutes and then rinsed most carefully. Interference with white counts and hemoglobin has frequently been reported after the use of household bleach (Domestos). The use of acid or alkali to remove protein is not recommended as the deposit may be charred and its removal may become even more difficult. However, no damage can be caused to the wafer even if the glass tube becomes etched.

The cause of a blockage may not always be obvious and may sometimes be the result of apparently insignificant changes. Latex particles, which replace white cells in some control preparations or may be used for calibration purposes, can cause build up and blockage, especially if the instrument is allowed to dry out. Neither bleach, acid, alkali, nor detergent will remove them. Rinsing the aperture tube in acetone may help in some circumstances but failing that, a low power ultrasonic bath, (not a probe) may be used for periods of up to a couple of seconds to loosen the blockage.

E. Excess aperture current will cause cell damage and electrothermal noise. The minimum setting which can be used conveniently should be chosen. A characteristic V-shaped vortex of warm electrolyte coming from the aperture, as seen on the aperture display, is typical of too high a setting.

F. When the instrument is clean and gives reproducible blood counts, with a background of less than 50 on the semi-automated systems, then it can be calibrated for cell counting.

WHITE CELL COUNTING

The white count is measured as the total number of nucleated cells present in a blood suspension at a 1:500 dilution. This suspension is prepared by lysing the red cells, which exceed the white cell numbers in normal fresh blood by approximately 1000:1. A size distribution curve should be established for a particular lytic agent and diluent in order to determine the correct counting conditions for that reagent. This counting plateau should be established using a fresh normal blood sample (see Note 2, p. 21). Any change in reagents will necessitate redetermination of this plateau position (see Note 3, p. 22). Do not use the white cells of a preserved control blood for this procedure as the size range of the white cells may be appreciably different from that of fresh blood.

White cell threshold calibration

The first step in counting white cells is to ensure that only cells of the appropriate size are counted. The instrument, usually the Coulter ® model ZF, should be fitted with a 100 μm aperture tube and 500 μl manometer. This instrument has automatic coincidence correction fitted and this should be turned on. If either another instrument or a 70 μm aperture are used, the instruction manual must be consulted. Alternative methods or tables for coincidence correction must also be used. Whatever the settings used, the white cells, prepared as below, should give a pulse height of 1½ to 2 cm on the monitor. The median pulse height — the position at which half the total white cell pulses can be excluded — should lie at between 25 and 35 threshold divisions. The current or attenuator settings may be increased or decreased one step if necessary to achieve this. Make a 1:500 dilution in electrolyte (40 μl blood plus 19.96 ml diluent), to produce at least 20 ml of dilution (see Hb note 2 and note 1 below) and add the correct quantity of lytic agent. The correct threshold settings should be determined by the method described in the manual. For the Coulter reagents Isoton® II and Zapoglobin® the correct WBC counting threshold for human blood is 35 ± 2 fl relative to red cell MCV calibration (q.v.).

Note 1

A 1:500 dilution is suitable for most normal and abnormal blood. Samples with high white counts, greater than 40 000/μl, should be diluted (perhaps a further 1:1) to give a raw count in the range of 8000 to 40 000. Coincidence correction must be applied to all counts above 10 000. Beware of carryover from high count specimens interfering with the next count. The Coulter® ZF and S family all make coincidence corrections automatically. Counts below $3 \times 10^9/l$ should be rechecked at a lower dilution such as 1:250.[11]

Note 2

Badly mixed samples will give erroneous results. This is especially likely with mixers where not every roller is driven. However, some clinical conditions can also give rise to apparently high white counts, for example:

1. Cold red-cell agglutinates may not be broken up by the lytic agent in the

time available. Warm the diluted blood to 37°C and use prediluted blood to overcome this if a Coulter S or similar apparatus is used.
2. Nucleated red cells will be counted with the white cells. If their numbers are significant a correction can be made but this will only be as accurate as the nucleated red cell count estimated from a blood film:

$$\text{Corrected WBC} = \frac{\text{WBC} - \text{WBC} \times \text{nucleated RBC}/100 \text{ WBC}}{100}$$

3. Cryoglobulin crystals,[12,13] cryofibrinogen[14] and crystalline hemoglobin have all been shown to register as 'white cells'. The first two can be eliminated by warming both diluent and samples as in (1) above; the latter is extremely rare.
4. Discrepant white cell counts have been reported for samples from patients with chronic leukemia, renal disease and those receiving cyclo-phosphamide therapy.[15] The cells in these patients are friable and the count will depend on the degree of fragmention caused by lytic agents as well as handling and mixing procedures.
5. Microbubbles, caused either by shaking a dilution, operating a diluter too violently, too rapid a transfer rate in automated instruments or too high a predilute vacuum sampling, will be counted as particles.
6. The use of silicone skin-wipes for finger-prick sampling can produce insoluble droplets of oil in the specimen. One unusual cause of a 'high white count' was an oily skin of a child who had been eating greasy food with its hands.[16]
7. The increased stroma content of cord bloods can give apparently high white cell counts if the threshold is mis-set, or if there is insufficient lytic agent.

Note 3

The instrument threshold settings are appropriate only for the lytic agent and diluent used for the calibration.
1. Some commercial lytic agents state that the white cells are stable for 30 minutes. This is not to be taken for granted. For example, with saponin the count will decrease steadily. This is because the cells continue to shrink and, as a result, fall below the counting threshold. Although the threshold can be re-set to give the same white count as by any other method, it may not do the same several minutes later and with different bloods. Some commercial reagents do not give a counting plateau.
2. Protein build-up will create an apparent increase in pulse height relative to the calibrated threshold setting. If the stroma pulse height exceeds this threshold, the count will rise. A partial blockage of the aperture by a tissue fibre or fibrin strand will have the same effect (see Note D, p. 20, cell counting and sizing).
3. A change of aperture tube even to one of similar nominal dimensions will require complete re-calibration.
4. Careless resetting or mishandling of the controls can alter instrument settings. This is not an uncommon cause of loss of accuracy.

Note 4

A background count should be the true background for the test vial, diluent, lytic agent and mixing technique. It should never exceed 2 per cent of the total cell count. High background counts may be the result of alkaline diluents attacking glass stock bottles. Lytic agents may also release particles from a vial wall or cap. Hard water, traces of detergent which interact with the lytic agent, as well as linen or paper wipe fibres left after washing vials may also increase the background count. Epithelial cells, transferred to the vial by placing the hand over the sample vial are a common cause of an increased background. Use only clean vials and clean caps for mixing. Whenever possible use them only once. The lytic agent itself may become a source of high background count unless the manufacturer's instructions are followed. If storage at room temperature is recommended, refrigeration could well form a countable precipitate and crystals may be formed in sunlight (see Hb Note 6).

Note 5

The calibration of the white cell count on a multiparameter automated cell counter may be performed by taking 10 fresh blood samples from normal subjects (Note Hb 8) and setting the average instrument result to that obtained by the reference method. These automated instruments are comparators, not absolute counters.

RED CELL COUNTING

The red cell count is generally taken to be the total count of cells with a volume greater than 25 fl in a balanced diluent. The enumention of red cells is closely related to estimating their size and these two aspects must be considered together. Setting the red cell count threshold to include all the cells of greater than 25 fl requires calibration of the instrument settings. This is fully described in the appropriate instruction manuals.

As with the white cell count, the reference method by which the red-cell count may be determined is basically simple. A whole blood sample should be accurately diluted to 1:50 000 in two stages in a particle-free balanced salt solution. The red-cells in suspension should then be counted using a properly calibrated single parameter analyzer such as the Coulter ZF.

Note 1

Poorly mixed samples will have a particularly marked effect on the red-cell count. Careful mixing between the two stages of dilution is essential (but not always achieved).

Note 2

The diluent used will control the cell volumes at the time the count is made. Although 0.9 per cent sodium chloride is considered isotonic, it will cause an immediate 10 per cent change of red cell volume followed by further size increases which may lead to cell rupture. Some reports suggest that K_3 EDTA

Table 2.1 Changes in the red cell count of a diluted (1: 50000) blood sample in different containers.

	Glass vial			Plastic vial		
Sample	0 min	30 min	% loss	0 min	30 min	% loss
1	2.95	2.80	5.1	2.95	2.74	7.1
2	2.68	2.58	3.7	2.68	2.46	8.6
3	5.49	5.19	5.5	5.49	5.27	9.4

gives unstable cell volumes which may increase up to 3 fl in four hours but this may have been due to the presence of a sorbate yeasticide. Filtered clean diluent solutions which are free of plasticisers (see Note 4) are commercially available and are strongly recommended for reference purposes.

Note 3

Cells may adhere to the wall of the counting vial and this may become significant at 1:50 000 dilution after 5 to 10 minutes. This phenomenon appears to be dependent on the material of the vial as well as the relative humidity which suggests that it may be a surface charge effect (Table 2.1). The cells are negatively charged and appear to migrate to the positively charged vessel wall. This is quite different from the fall in the measured count caused by repeatedly counting the same diluted sample. Here, the passage of current through the suspension of cells in electrolyte can have three effects. Firstly, the current appears to affect the red cell enzymes, paralyzing the sodium pump mechanism and allowing the cell to swell slowly. Secondly, the release of chloride ions at the anode will affect the cell surface. Thirdly, a tonicity gradient can be set up through the electrolyte with the result that some cells will swell and burst, thereby diminishing the count. Once a sample has been counted the changes will commence and after five minutes the sample should be discarded. A further sub-sample, from a stock not exposed to current, should be used if multiple counts are required. The red cells in the master stock will remain within 1 per cent of their original volume for at least 30 minutes and possibly for up to two hours[17].

Note 4

Lytic agents and plasticisers are known to affect the red cell count and size.[18,19,20] They will, moreover, have different effects on fresh and preserved red cells and this is particularly important in calibrating automated multichannel analyzers such as the Coulter S.
1. Plasticizers are organic chemicals, usually high esters such as dioctylphthalate, which are interspaced between polymer molecules and allow them to move in relation to one another. They can leach into diluter flow lines and markedly affect the red cell size and count in fresh blood samples. Preserved whole blood materials are much less readily affected by solubilized plasticizers and calibration with such materials will lead to erroneous results for fresh samples in the presence of such contamination.
2. The presence of plasticizers can be detected by comparing the cell volume from the suspect automated method with that of a contaminant free dilution.

Take an unopened container of diluent. Pour, do not pipette or use a potentially contaminated tap, approximately 20 ml of the diluent into a brand new counting vial. Add 0.2 to 0.4 μl fresh blood, using a wooden applicator or new piece of fuse wire, to give a count of 50 to 100 × 10^6/l. The cell volume of this suspension should then be compared with that recorded by the automated system for the same blood sample. The difference should be no more than 2 fl. Plasticizer or lytic agent contamination will often raise the cell volume by 5 to 15 fl.

3. The source of the contamination may simply be lytic agent absorbed onto protein bound around the aperture or trapped behind rubber bands unwisely used for holding electrodes in place. Detergents remaining in sample vials or caps after they have been washed is an extremely common finding. Traces of lytic agent on the hands that replace diluent input tubing when a new diluent supply is connected will also cause similar errors. Plasticizers are more difficult to trace and PVC tubing used on some diluters must be suspected. Reagent stock bottles should be unplasticized high or medium density polyethylene. Flow lines should be made of high density polyethylene tubing or silicone rubber which is free of plasticizer effects.

HEMATOCRIT AND MEAN CELL VOLUME

The hematocrit or packed cell volume can be estimated by two techniques. The reference technique is based on the microhematocrit. The commonly used electrical impedance method can show good correlation with this,[21] but there can be important differences.[22] A 3 per cent difference has been attributed to plasma trapped amongst red cell in the microhematocrit method.[23] However, earlier work suggests that this might account for only 1 per cent of the difference.[24] It seems likely that the method used to measure trapped plasma[25] may have been substantially influenced by albumin coating the red cells.[26,27] The value of an empirical 'correction' for plasma trapping in the calculation of MCV seems doubtful.

The microhematocrit should be measured in six tubes which have been nearly filled with fresh whole blood by centrifuging at $10-13 \times 10^3$ g at 20°C for five minutes. EDTA in excess of 2 mg/ml blood will cause osmotic shrinkage[28] and must be avoided. The proportion of the whole column of blood occupied by red cells should be read using a microscope with a moving stage and vernier scale.[29] The MCV may then be calculated by dividing (PCV × 1000) by the red cell count.

Calibration of electronic methods of estimating MCV must be carried out by first calculating the MCV for at least 10 properly anticoagulated fresh blood samples. The mean reference MCV is calculated from accurate measurements of the red cell count and PCV by the reference techniques. The mean result from the instrument for the same samples should be adjusted to equal the mean result obtained by the reference methods.

The choice of samples for calibration should exclude those conditions which have been shown to alter the size of the red cell in the measuring system. Cold agglutinates which increase MCV^2 can be quite common and high white cell counts in the presence of low red cell counts can also cause MCV changes[30] as can antibodies coating the red cells.[31]

Automated hematocrit
In the Coulter family of automated cell counters the hematocrit is calculated from the red cell count and the mean cell volume. The red cell count used is derived in a separate counting circuit from the RBC and may differ from this by up to 0.5 per cent. This hematocrit must not be equated with the spun hematocrit. It must not be calibrated by setting it equal to the value given for a blood sample or control preparation but must be set to equal the product of red cell count and mean cell volume obtained divided by 1000 on any one fresh blood. A useful check of the accuracy of the arithmetic is to ensure that:

$$\frac{MCV \times RBC}{Hct} = 1000 \pm 30$$

This check can readily be carried out for all samples by on-line monitoring of the data.

Mean cell hemoglobin (MCH)
This parameter is largely the offspring of automated cell counting. It is calculated as $\frac{Hb \times 10}{RBC}$. As with the hematocrit its calibration must not be based on the given values for a control preparation. It must be set equal to the value calculated from the hemoglobin concentration and red cell count. The multiplication factor may be checked by ensuring that:

$$\frac{RBC}{Hb} \times MCH = 10 \pm 0.30$$

Mean cell hemoglobin concentration (MCHC)
In automated electronic cell counters this is calculated from all three directly measured red cell parameters:

$$MCHC = \frac{Hb \times 1000}{Rbc \times MCV}$$

Again, this parameter must not be calibrated by setting it equal to a given value for a blood sample or control preparation, however that result may have been derived. To maintain the internal consistency of the automated apparatus the MCHC should be set equal to the value calculated from the primary measurements, preferably on a fresh blood sample. The accuracy of the arithmetic involved can be checked by ensuring that:

$$\frac{RBC \times MCV}{Hb} \times MCHC = 1000 \pm 30$$

PLATELETS

The reference technique for platelet counting is still hemocytometry using a counting chamber. The large coefficients of variation inherent in the relatively low numbers of platelets counted in this technique have stimulated the use of electronic cell counters. There may be a systematic difference between the two techniques in that some electronic methods do not cover the full pathological range of platelet sizes. In methods that depend upon separation of platelets from red cells, the variability of the processes involved and the need to make a possibly inappropriate hematocrit correction give rise to many errors. This is often compounded by a lack of understanding of proper instrument calibration. In addition, platelet control preparations usually have a different size distribution to fresh platelets. All these factors have contributed towards the poor standardization of platelet counts.[32]

Reference method for platelet counting by hemocytometry[60]
1. Blood specimens should be anticoagulated with EDTA at 1.5 to 2.0 mg/ml and should be no more than four hours old.
2. Counting chambers should be of the Neubauer design and conform to the appropriate national standard (e.g. BS 748) such that the accuracy of the volume is better than ± 1 per cent.
3. The diluting fluid should be 1 per cent ammonium oxalate prepared from analytical grade reagent dissolved in deionized water and filtered through a 0.22 μm membrane filter, stored at 4°C until used.
4. The pipettes used should be certified to better than 1 per cent for small volumes and grade A for larger volumes.
5. A 1:20 dilution of freshly mixed blood in ammonium oxalate solution should be prepared by adding 100 μl to 1.9 ml diluent in a 75 × 12 mm tube. This should be mixed for 10 minutes.
6. Two such dilutions should be used to fill two counting chambers each and these left to settle in a moist atmosphere for 20 minutes. The chambers should be counted on a phase contrast microscope at × 100 magnification. At least 500 platelets should be counted. Photography of the counting chamber to allow more than one operator to count the bright refractile objects on enlargements can help eliminate observer error. While errors in this count can be minimized by this reference method the accuracy is limited by the number of cells counted. For a total of 500 platelets the coefficient of variation will be 5 per cent. At a platelet count of $150 \times 10^9/l$ the 95 per cent confidence limits within which the true results may lie will be $135-165 \times 10^9/l$.

Electronic platelet counting
There are two different approaches and each may have its own problems. One method involves counting particles of a predetermined size in a diluted sample of whole blood (e.g. Coulter S Plus and Ultraflo 100). The older and as yet more common method, involves counting particles in a suspension derived from platelet rich plasma. Provided that the counter is correctly set and will count particles with a volume between 3 and 36 fl there is little difficulty in simply enumerating the particles in the platelet rich suspension. The main difficulties arise in preparing such a suspension and it seems unlikely that any method will be perfect. Instruments using whole blood platelet counting have recently be-

come more common but as yet there is no primary method for their calibration. All the methods, be they based on dilution in urea to obtain transparent red cells or based on platelet size distribution, depend on an instrument which is basically a comparator. As with other such automated equipment calibration is indirect. That is, a value must first be ascribed to a series of whole blood samples by the reference method and the automated platelet counter then set so that it will give the same values when presented with these specimens.

Note 1

The original measurements of platelet volume were based on apparatus calibrated by reference to blood containing red cells with a volume calculated from the red cell count and hematocrit. The range usually seen is 3 to 30 fl using this red cell based scale although occasionally platelets may be much larger. Platelet counting apparatus is usually set to cover the range 3 to 36 fl. Recently, latex spheres in the volume range of 4 or 13 fl have become available and may be used to calibrate platelet counters. The scale will however be different and platelets in the range of 3 to 36 fl, as defined by the red cell volume, would have a volume of 2 to 24 fl on a latex scale. The technique for calibration using red cells is described.

1. Blood containing red cells of known mean cell volume (in the region 85 to 95 fl) should be used.
2. Prepare a 1: 50 000 dilution using a clean source of diluent and clean counting vial to exclude volume changes.
3. Using an instrument fitted with a 70 μm aperture tube, with the coincidence correction off, and a 0.1 ml manometer to limit the count time, take a series of counts as described. Calculate the calibration factor.
   Example: Coulter Counter ZF; for red cell counting the settings may be attenuation = 4, aperture current = 8, half count at threshold 25.5 for a blood of MCV 84 femtolitres (the different settings here for the red count are due to the aperture tube size being different.
   a. If the total average red cell count is 9133 (ignoring coincidence correction) then the half count = 4566.
   b. Taking counts at increasing thresholds about the median gives:

Threshold	Counts
22	7225
24	5858
25	5249
25.5	4676
26	4306

   The half count of the blood is therefore at threshold 25.5 (within 0.5 division).
   c. The threshold factor = $\dfrac{\text{MCV}}{\text{half count threshold}} = \dfrac{84}{25.5}$
4. The pulse height on the oscilloscope should now be increased by three

doubling steps using the attenuator switch, i.e. from A = 4 to A = 0.5. This represents an eightfold increase in amplification. The calibration factor now becomes $\frac{3.294}{8}$ = 0.412 fl/threshold division. The threshold corresponding to 3 fl is therefore $\frac{3}{0.412}$ = 7.3 divisions. The upper threshold would be = 87 divisions. It may be necessary to alter the attenuation settings one step either way such that the lower threshold lies between 5 and 9 to avoid counting 'noise' and so that the upper threshold does not exceed 100. Thrombo-counter® instruments have built in circuitry that duplicates this calibration procedure.

Note 2
Specimen quality will determine the quality of the results for platelet counting. EDTA, as either the sodium or potassium salt, is the only anti-coagulant which will preserve platelets for up to four hours. Platelet aggregation and count loss as a result of the presence of platelet antibodies or EDTA mediated agglutinating factors may be less likely to be noticed in automated methodologies.[34,35,36] Citrate will reduce the platelet count by 20 per cent in two minutes.[70] Apparatus which does not allow large platelets (> 36 fl) to be counted will underestimate the platelet count, particularly in Mediterranean areas.[37]

Note 3
Platelet reference materials are readily available but the particles are usually much smaller than fresh blood platelets[33] (Fig. 2.3) and a proportion may fall below the lower threshold for most automated systems. Marginal alteration or maladjustments of the critical lower threshold, whilst having little or no effect on fresh blood platelet counts, will produce large changes in the count for such reference materials. Even a preparation which perfectly matched the real distribution would include 'platelet dust' or cellular debris. Lowering both upper and lower threshold could give the specified assay value for the material but still underestimate the platelet count of fresh blood. Such materials cannot be used as calibrators.

Note 4
Background counts should be less than 1 per cent of the total count. Because of the smaller volume range covered, more critical control of background is required than for red or white cell counting. Bacterial contamination in diluents can reach levels in warm weather where the bacteriostat is no longer sufficient. Aggregates of these bacteria may then move into the counting range. Sterilization may be necessary to restore a low background. Increasing preservative levels can cause cell damage and is not advisable. Washed vials may appear clean but can shed platelet-sized material and increase background. In addition the dangers of lytic agents and plasticizers (see red cells Note 4), p. 24 apply equally to platelet counting.

Note 5
Dilution of platelet rich plasma should be made with great care. If red cells are

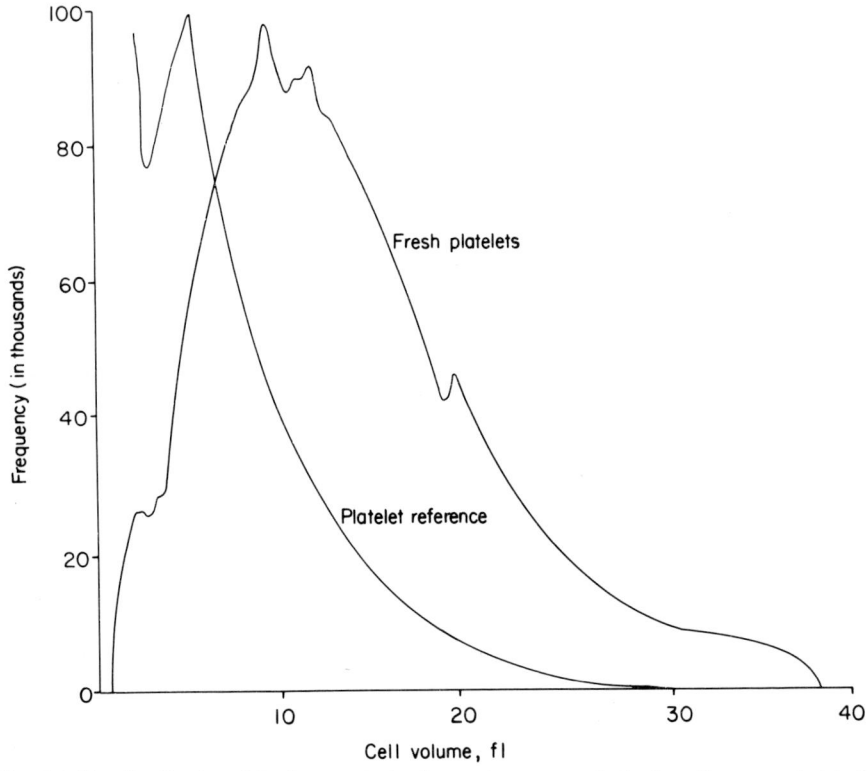

Fig. 2.3 Size distribution of fresh normal platelets and a preserved platelet reference material. The cell volume has been calibrated by reference to red cells whose volume had been calculated from RBC and hematocrit. Calibration against latex particles would give a scale with incremental points at 7, 14, 21 and 28 fl.

present in excessive numbers they may mask platelets and give rise to erroneously low results. Red cells should not exceed 15 per cent of the total platelet count[38] and no more than 1000 particles should be counted above the upper threshold. This caveat does not, of course, apply to whole blood platelet counters employing hydrodynamic focusing and one-by-one cell sizing techniques. For any cell counting procedure the numbers counted should be large enough to ensure adequate precision. Electronic counts should lie between 8000 and 24 000 to be in the best range for precision without increasing coincidence beyond the limits of the correction formulae. If necessary the dilution should be adjusted to achieve this. The computation of results presents a large area for potential error but full understanding of the mechanism of the method will eliminate it. Even marginal deviations from a recommended method should be discussed with instrument manufacturers to ensure that the calculations are valid for each and every factor present.

THE USE OF ELECTRONIC PULSES FOR CALIBRATION

Pulse generators are available for checking electronic circuitry in cell counting apparatus. The circuits checked are usually the preamplifier, amplifier threshold and output circuits. This can have value in verifying that the electronic calibration has not changed. However, none of these checks include the aperture current, nor can they detect the sensing zone changes which occur as a result of blockage, protein build up, or variation in vacuum. For semi-automated counters the sample counted depends on a fixed volume of fluid drawn through the aperture. Temperature variations will affect the flow rate and frequency-dependent pulses are of little value in detecting these. The pulse shapes created by cells passing through such apertures will be complex and varied. The cell counter circuits are designed to accept these 'natural' pulses. Simulated signals should produce similarly shaped pulses to give a valid comparison. Constant square wave pulse forms would give totally misleading information.

CALIBRATION OF CELL SIZE DISTRIBUTION

There are occasions when for one reason or another the laboratory may wish to measure the size distribution of either red cells, white cells or platelets. Latex particles in suspension with carefully defined mean volumes may then be used to calibrate volume discriminators or scales. However, the apparently simple physical characteristics of these preparations can become complicated during analysis. They can form aggregates whose size may depend on their age and degree of dispersion. Although detergents may be included in the suspension their effect can be over-ridden by age. In addition, it is not always clear by which average measure the volume of the latex particles has been defined. If the mean volume has been used then calibration will be dependent upon the degree of aggregation of the suspension presented to the counting apparatus. The mode can only be readily determined by multi-channel analysis and it is not always applicable to blood counting apparatus. The median has the advantage that it is least affected by aggregation and can, with care, be determined on blood counters.

Whether it is the mean, median or mode that is specified this must always refer to the singlet particle population so that aggregated polymers are excluded from consideration. It is important therefore to determine from the supplier of the material which characteristic is specified and to follow the manufacturer's instructions to define this specified point in the distribution.

The volume attributed to latex particles is defined by physical measurements such as scanning electronmicroscopy and Stoke's Law sedimentation coefficients. Red cell size on the other hand is derived from the red cell count and the hematocrit. There seem to be considerable differences in the volumes that may be attributed to red cells by these two definitions. Red cells with a mean volume of 85 fl calculated from the red cell count and hematocrit would, when measured on an instrument calibrated with latex, appear to have a volume of only 63 fl. The reason for this difference is not clear although it may be related to the elasticity of the red cell membrane compared with the absolute rigidity of the latex particle. It is essential, therefore, to specify which scale of calibration is used in any expression of cell size distribution. A more practical, but nevertheless important, point is that some latex suspension contain detergents. These are added to prevent latex aggregation but may also be carried over into subsequent samples and interfere with the measurement of the MCV and red cell count in fresh blood samples. The scale by which volume is measured is only as accurate as the assumptions made for the calibrating material.

The properties of embalmed semi-preserved bloods have been discussed in relation to their role as controls. Fixed cells could also be useful for MCV calibration in different diluents if their mean volume changed as the electrolyte changed and they showed the same osmotic response as fresh red cells. Similarly a stable suspension of cells would be valuable if they showed no aggregation.

A perfect calibrator would lift the burden of calibration with fresh blood from often overworked laboratories. It would simplify the calibration procedure and lead to better inter-laboratory control. However very stable cell suspensions may, by definition, be unaffected by diluents of differing osmotic pressure or even the presence of plasticizer. It follows that care must always be exercised with the use of any so called calibrator. Their very stability makes them different from the real cells with which hematology is concerned.

REFERENCES

1. International Committee for Standardization in Hematology, 1978. Recommendations for reference method for hemoglobinometry in human blood (ICSH Standard EP6/2: 1977) and specifications for international hemiglobincyanide reference preparation (ICSH Standard EP6/3: 1977) Journal of Clinical Pathology 31: 139–143
2. Hattersley P G, Gerard P W, Caggiano V, Nash D R 1971 Erroneous values on the Model S Coulter Counter due to high titer cold autoagglutinins. American Journal of Clinical Pathology 55: 442–446
3. Nicholls P D 1973 Erroneous Model S Coulter Counter values on patients undergoing parenteral nutrition with iintravenous lipid emulsions. Medical Laboratory Technology. 30: 293–295
4. Nosanchuk J S, Roark M F, Wanser C 1974 Anemia masked by triglyceridemia. American Journal of Clinical Pathology. 62: 838–839
5. Gagne C, Auger P L, Moorjani S, Brun D, Lupien J P 1977 Effect of hyperchylomicronemia on the measurement of hemoglobin. American Journal of Clinical Pathology. 68: 584–586
6. Mahr G, 1974 Hämoglobinbestimmung bei Morbus Waldenstrom. Deutsche Medizinische Wochenschrift 33: 1665–1666
7. Eichen S, Mandel J, Schwerk R D, Warfield D L 1977 Accurate hemoglobin determination. American Journal of Clinical Pathology 68: 91–92
8. Salvati A M, Samoggia P, Taggi F, Tentori L 1977 Hemoglobinometry: A comparison between the hemiglobincyanide method and the Coulter S Counter. Clinica Chimica Acta 77: 13–20
9. Koepke J A, 1977 The calibration of automated instruments for accuracy in hemoglobinometry. American Journal of Clinical Pathology 68: 180–184
10. Koepke J A, Bull B S, Gilmer P R Jr, Goldblatt S A 1978 Hematology In: Inhorn S L (ed) Quality Assurance Practices for Health Laboratories. American Public Health Association, New York, p 687–744
11. Hurd K E, Palmer M K Hull S 1977 A comparative study for the enumeration of peripheral blood white cell counts below $2.0 \times 10^9/l$ using counting chambers and the Coulter Counter Model 'S'. Journal of Clinical Pathology 30: 1005–1006
12. Gulliani G L, Hyun B H, Gabaldon H 1977 Falsely elevated automated leukocyte counts on cryoglobulinemic and/or cryofibrinogenemic blood samples. Laboratory Medicine 8: 14–26
13. Abela M, McArdle B Qureshi M 1980 Pseudoleucocytosis due to cryoglobulinemia. Journal of Clinical Pathology 33: 796
14. Smith S B, Arkin C 1972 Cryofibrinogenemia. Incidence, clinical correlations, and a review of literature. American Journal of Clinical Pathology 58: 524–530
15. Luke R G Koepke J A, Siegel R R 1971 The effects of immuno-suppressive drugs and uremia on automated leukocyte counts. American Journal of Clinical Pathology 56: 503–507

16. Ratcliffe J 1976 Blood count discrepancies. Medical Laboratory Sciences 33: 475
17. Lawrence A C K, Bevington J M, Young M 1975 Storage of blood and the mean corpuscular volume. Journal of Clinical Pathology 28: 345–349
18. Young M, Lawrence A C K, Bevington J M, Young M 1975 The influence of extraneous factors on Coulter S measurement of the mean corpuscular volume. Journal of Clinical Pathology 28: 12–15
19. Lewis S M, Stoddart C T H 1971 Effects of anticoagulants and containers (glass and plastic) on the blood count. Laboratory Practise 10: 787–792
20. Richards R J, Desai R, Rose F A 1976 A surface-active agent involved in PVC-induced hemolysis. Nature 260: 53–54
21. Penn D, Williams P R, Dutcher T F, Adair R M 1979 Comparison of hematocrit determinations by microhematrocrit and electronic particle counter. American Journal of Clinical Pathology 72: 71–74
22. Fairbanks V F, 1980 Nonequivalence of automated and manual hematocrit and erythrocytic indices. American Journal of Clinical Pathology 73: 55–62
23. England J M, Walford D M, Waters D A W 1972 Reassessment of the reliability of the hematocrit. British Journal of Hematology 23: 247–256
24. Garby I, Vuille J C, 1961 The amount of trapped plasma in a high speed micro-capillary hematocrit centrifuge. Scandinavian Journal of Clinic and Laboratory Investigation 13: 642–645
25. England J M, Down M C 1975 Determination of the packed cell volume using ^{131}I-Human Serum Albumin 30: 365–370
26. Hughes-Jones N C, Gardner B 1962 The exchange of 131 I-labelled protein between red cells and serum. Biochemical Journal 83: 404–412
27. Jay A W L 1975 Geometry of the human erythrocyte. Biophysical Journal 15: 205–222
28. Brittin G M, Brecher G, Johnson C A 1969 Elimination of error in hematocrit produced by excessive EDTA. American Journal of Clinical Pathology 52: 780–783
29. Crosland-Taylor P J, Allen R W B, England J M, Fielding J F, Lewis S M, Shinton N K, White J M 1979 Draft protocol for testing calibration and qualifity control material used with automatic blood-counting apparatus. Clinical and Laboratory Haematology1: 61–64
30. Levick G M, Hudson M J 1977 Erroneous MCV results with a Coulter 'S' Medical Laboratory Sciences 34: 179
31. Brittin G M, Brecher G, Johnson C, Stuart J 1969 Spurious macrocytosis of antibody-coated red cells. American Journal of Clinical Pathology 52: 237–241
32. Wertz R K, Koepke J A 1977 A critical analysis of platelet counting methods. American Journal of Clinical Pathoogy 68: 195–201
33. Lewis S M, Wardle J, Cousins S, Skelly J V 1979 Platelet counting-development of a reference method and a reference preparation. Clinical and Laboratory Hematology 1: 227–237
34. Kjeldsberg C R, Hershgold E J 1974 Spurious thrombocytopenia. Journal of American Medical Association 227: 628–630
35. Mant M J, Doery J C G, Gauldie J, Sims H 1975 Pseudothrombocytopenia due to platelet aggregion and degranulation in blood collected in EDTA. Scandinavian Journal of Hematology 15: 161–170
36. Schreiner D P, Bell W R 1973 Pseudothrombocytopenia: Manifestation of a new type of platelet agglutinin. Blood 42: 541–549
37. von Behrens W E 1975 Mediterranean macrothrombocytopenia. Blood 46: 199–208
38. Maxie M G 1977 Evaluation of techniques for counting bovine platelets. Canadian Journal of Comparative Medicine 41: 409–415

3
Quality Assurance and Standardization in Blood Group Serology
A. M. Holburn

Quality assurance schemes for blood group serology do not yet match the sophistication and reliability of the schemes now applied in clinical chemistry or other parts of hematology. Serological tests are at best semi-quantitative and quality assurance schemes have been much less rapidly applied in these circumstances. Indeed, a case has been made for the application to serology of the concept of 'zero defects'. This is a system for quality assurance that has been applied in the aerospace industry[1,2] in which a product, such as a space vehicle, cannot be test flown and must therefore function perfectly first time. Perfect function is guaranteed by sound design and by the elimination of all defects in each component of the product. Defects are eliminated by the application of rigid quality control procedures at every stage of construction. By analogy, the final product of blood banking, a transfusion of blood, cannot be tested and must also be right first time.

Rigid quality control can be applied to the equipment and reagents used in serological tests but, in order to achieve zero defects, the accuracy and precision of procedures that make up each component part of serological tests must also be defined. This information is, however, extremely scarce.[3] Lack of precision is inherent in the use, traditional in blood group serology, of such semi-quantitative procedures as assessment of cell concentration by eye and of volumes by drop counting.[4] The performer of the tests who must make subjective assessments of the results and put interpretations upon them is even less susceptible to the application of rigid quality control. Thus the strict application of the concept of zero defects to blood banking must await the introduction of a much greater degree of automation into serological methods particularly in the reading and interpretation of patterns of results.

Accuracy in blood group serology is probably best assessed in terms of error rates. Within the laboratory, clerical and technical error rates can be measured by careful and regular scrutiny of laboratory records and by the maintenance of a register of such errors as are known to have occurred. There are only a few reports documenting the incidence of errors in blood banks. In one study 12 technical and 52 clerical errors were recorded over a 21 month period during which 5806 transfusions were given,[5] and in another 46 technical and 33 clerical errors were recorded in the collection, processing and crossmatching of blood over a two year period.[6] More recently, an American group reported 24 technical and 101 clerical errors over a two-year period, an incidence of one error per 500 units of blood transfused.[7] In an attempt to determine the true error rate the latter group introduced a system of performance evaluation wherein discrepant data were deliberately introduced into various areas of the laboratory. The rate of failure to detect these errors depended on the area of work and showed an improvement in the course of time but over a four year period 11 per cent of errors remained undetected.[8] It must be assumed that at least 11 per cent of real errors can remain undetected and that, in other laboratories, with a lower level of consciousness of the problem, an even higher proportion of errors may go undetected. Following their investigations this same group recently designed a functional classification of errors which included the categories of identification, performance, interpretation, transcription and filing. In their experience transcription and filing errors accounted for 93.7 per cent of errors.[9]

EXTERNAL PROFICIENCY TESTING PROGRAMS

Accuracy or error rates can be estimated by formal proficiency tests. Two groups, the College of American Pathologists (CAP) and the Ontario Medical Association (OMA) have published results of proficiency assessments. National schemes have also been established in Australia, New Zealand, the United Kingdom and in Belgium. There are considerable variations in the design of these schemes and in the calculation and reporting of error rates. It is, therefore, difficult to compare the results from different countries but it is clear that serious errors are relatively commonplace and that they extend even to simple ABO and Rh grouping.

Uncomplicated ABO amd Rh(D) Grouping

The error rates observed in the CAP program for uncomplicated ABO and Rh(D) grouping have appeared in a series of publicatons[10-16] and are summarized in Table 3.1. Since 1974 a combined error rate has been reported for ABO and Rh(D) grouping. There has been little improvement over recent years. The results of these surveys are normally expressed as rates of concurrence between

Table 3.1 Error rates for uncomplicated ABO and Rh(D) grouping (College of American Pathologists).

Year	Errors per 100 Participants	
	ABO	Rh(D)
1964	4.3	
1966	9.0	
1967	2.6	2.4
1968	0.9–5.6	0.9–3.6
1969	0.8–2.4	0.8–2.4
1973	0.7	1.3
	ABO and Rh(D)	
1974	0.1–0.9	
1975	0.3–1.6	
1976	0.6–3.4	
1977	0.6–5.1	

participants and a selected group of reference laboratories. A continued concurrence of 94 per cent or better in ABO and Rh(D) testing has been observed and from this it has been concluded that participants have achieved a 'high and stable level of excellency'.[16] Commenting on performance in the CAP program, Weiner emphasized that in ABO and Rh(D) grouping nothing short of perfection is acceptable and that little comfort is to be drawn from these results.[17]

In the CAP program failure to enter a result is treated as an error. In 1975 5.7 per cent to 84 per cent of all ABO and Rh(D) errors were due to failure to record results and comparable numbers of failures were reported for 1976. The view has been expressed that many of the other errors in simple ABO and Rh(D) grouping revealed in the CAP program are also clerical in origin, if only because it is so difficult to accept that there are laboratories in which routine ABO and Rh(D) grouping is not performed reliably.[14,18] In the United States, reagents released by manufacturers must satisfy rigid requirements for potency and specificity.[19] Technical failures would necessarily be the result of gross incompetence and misuse of reagent controls. In an attempt to confirm the belief that most errors were of clerical origin the organizers of the CAP program asked each participant that recorded an ABO or Rh(D) error to check the original work-sheet. Far from confirming the organizers' faith, the replies of most participants implied that they must have received the wrong sample since the laboratory in question did not make errors.[14,20] While it is certain that clerical errors are important, one cannot escape the conclusion that technical errors may be equally important.

The Centre for Disease Control (CDC), Atlanta, monitors performance in laboratories in the United States on behalf of the US Department of Health, Education and Welfare. The CDC reports its results as the per cent of laboratories returning unacceptable results (Table 3.2).[21] Most errors in ABO grouping were of subgrouping or non-reporting. Major errors in ABO grouping which could have had serious consequence in clinical situations have, however, also been observed and there has been no evidence of improvement in recent years.

Table 3.2 Error rates for uncomplicated ABO and Rh(D) grouping (Centre for Disease Control).

Year	Percent of laboratories reporting unacceptable results ABO	Rh(D)
1977	0.5–13.1	0.6–5.5
1978	0.2–22.5	0.6–7.8
1979	0.3–13.6	0.7–6.3

The OMA has reported error rates in uncomplicated ABO grouping in terms of errors per 1000 opportunities for error (Table 3.3).[22,23] The error rates in Ontario have not changed over the four years 1975 to 1979 and the organizers of this program believe that these rates may represent an irreducible minimum of clerical and technical errors.[23] The error rates for uncomplicated Rh(D) grouping have improved significantly over the period of the survey but the rate remains higher than that for ABO grouping. It is unlikely that the reporting of Rh(D) grouping is more prone to clerical error than reporting of ABO grouping. These error rates therefore tend to confirm the suspicion that technical errors occur, at least in simple Rh(D) grouping.

Table 3.3 Error rates for uncomplicated ABO and Rh(D) grouping (Ontario Medical Association).

Year	Errors per 1000 Opportunities ABO	Rh(D)
1975–1977	1.3	6.6
1977–1979	1.4	2.3
		$p < 0.001$

Complicated ABO and Rh(D) grouping

The error rates detected for complicated ABO and Rh(D) grouping tests have been very much worse than for uncomplicated grouping. In two CAP surveys, a group A_2 or A_2B blood with a potent anti-A_1 has been issued. In 1966 26 per cent of participants failed to report accurately the A_2 subgroup[11] and the results were no better in 1977 when 41.4 per cent failed to report accurately the A_2B group and only 39 per cent of those who would normally be expected to be able to do so, identified the accompanying antibody as anti-A_1.[16] The effect on ABO grouping of a positive direct antiglobulin test was investigated in CAP surveys in 1973[12] and 1974.[13] In 1973 group A, Rh(D)-positive cells which were coated with anti-D were misgrouped as AB by 13.5 per cent of participants. It was suggested that the positive reactions of these coated cells with anti-B reagents may have been due to the inclusion of additives in commercial reagents. In 1974 group Rh(D)-positive cells weakly coated with anti-c were issued. These cells were misgrouped as A or A_2 12 times, an error rate of 0.56 per cent. This was a marked improvement but the cells were only weakly coated.

The experience of the OMA has been similar. Complicated problems of ABO and Rh(D) grouping are associated with increased error rates and in addition there has been no evidence of improvement over the period 1975 to 1979. A group O cell with a missing alloantibody has been issued in three OMA surveys. The error rate in ABO grouping of these cells varied from 0 to 10.7 per 1000 opportunities and the missing anti-B was 'detected' 32 to 196 times per 1000 opportunities. Group A_2 or A_2B cells accompanied by strong anti-A_1 have been issued on three occasions. The error rate in ABO grouping of these cells varied from 3.7 to 21.4 per 1000 opportunities and the anti-A_1 was missed on 45 to 189 occasions per 1000 opportunities. In two surveys samples were issued containing mixtures of group O and A cells, simulating the blood of a group A patient who had received a transfusion of group O blood. The error rates in ABO grouping of these cells were 24.8 and 15.3 per 1000 opportunities but the mixed field reaction was missed on 920 and 650 occasions per 1000 opportunities. Very poor performance in the detection of mixed field agglutination has been reported by others.[4] Group O T-activated cells issued in an OMA survey in 1978 were grouped as A or AB by 15.4 per cent of participants and a further

31.2 per cent did not offer an interpretation of the ABO blood group. Only 53.4 per cent correctly identified the T-activated cells as group O. On three occasions the OMA have investigated the error rates in complicated Rh(D) grouping. Group Rh(D)-negative cells strongly coated with IgG antibody have been issued three times. In the first of these surveys the cells were reported as Rh(D)-positive on nearly one third of possible opportunities; the results have since improved significantly but the error rate remains above 5 per cent of opportunities (Table 3.4).

Table 3.4 Errors rates for complicated Rh(D) grouping (Ontario Medical Association).

Problem	Year	Error	Error per 1000 Opportunities
Rh(D)–negative cells with strong positive DAGT	1977 1978 1979	Interpreted as Rh(D) -positive	306 82 57

Direct antiglobulin test

In the 1973 CAP survey cells were issued which were strongly coated with anti-D.[12] This produced a 13.5 per cent error in ABO grouping but participants were not asked to record results of direct antiglobulin testing. In the 1974 CAP survey, cells weakly (1+) sensitized with anti-c were issued and on the report form a space was also provided for the result of antiglobulin testing. The error rate in ABO grouping fell to 0.56 per cent but 12.8 per cent of participants reported a negative direct antiglobulin test for these cells. No correlation was found between performance and manufacture of antiglobulin reagent. In the 1977 CAP survey cells strongly sensitized (3 to 4+) with anti-D were issued.[16] Only 0.1 per cent of participants recorded negative results for direct antiglobulin tests but 13.7 per cent recorded weak (1 to 2+) reactions.

Table 3.5 Error rates in direct antiglobulin test (Ontario Medical Association).

Year	Cell coating	Error per 1000 opportunities
1976	IgG	50.4
1977	C	40.0
1977	IgG	17.2
1978	IgG	4.0
1978	IgG	6.5
1979	IgG	4.2

In the OMA program cells strongly coated (3 to 4) with IgG or complement have been issued in six surveys between 1976 and 1979.[23] The error rates are given in Table 3.5. There has been a notable improvement in performance in direct antiglobulin testing over the period of observation.

Antibody detection and identification

Since 1975 performance in the CAP program has been analyzed on the basis of

Table 3.6 Error rates for antibody detection and identification (College of American Pathologists).

Year	Antibody	Errors per 100 participants Detection	Detection and identification
1973	$-P_1$	28.0	38.0
	$-e$	0.4	2.3
	$-K$	0.2	0.7
1974	$-E$	6.1	19.6
	$-C + D$	0.2	1.8
	$-e + Ce$	0.1	10.1
1975	$-k$	1.8	35.0
	$-I$	11.7	
	$-Le^a$	42.5	
	$Fy^a + K$	3.4	8.5
1976	$-D$	0.2	
	$-S$	53	
	$-c$	4.0	
	$-K$	0.2	
1977	$-c$	3.7	4.0
	$-A_1 + Lu^b$	8.9	A_1 61.0
			Lu^b 70.6
	$-C + D$	1.9	1.8

the extent of services offered by the participating laboratory. The extent of services has been defined as
1. ABO and Rh(D) grouping only.
2. ABO and Rh(D) grouping and irregular antibody detection.
3. ABO and Rh(D) grouping, irregular antibody detection and identification.

The error rates for extent 2 laboratories (antibody detection) and for extent 3 laboratories (antibody detection and identification) are given in Table 3.6. Antibody detection is considered to be at very good levels of acccuracy. Poor results were, however, obtained with several antibodies, an anti-P_1 which was only weakly reactive at room temperature, a weak anti-Lewis and a very weak anti-S.

Table 3.7 Error rates in antibody detection and identification (Centre for Disease Control).

Year	Antibody	Percent of laboratories reporting unacceptable results Detection	Identification
1977	$-K$	3.2	5.8
	$-Fy^a$	3.2	10.1
	$-c$	3.3	16.3
	$-E + c + S$	4.2	37.3
1978	$-D + Fy^a$	3.6	17.2
	$-K$	4.1	1.7
	$-E$	5.5	4.6
1979	$-C$	6.6	16.8
	$-Fy^a$	24.5	14.8

There is no evident trend towards improvement in antibody detection in the CAP surveys but the antibodies issued have varied in specificity and in potency. On the present results it is clear that some potent antibodies are not being detected and these include as many as 4 per cent of Rh antibodies. Very recently similar results have been reported by the Centre for Disease Control (Table 3.7).[21]

The results for antibody detection obtained in the surveys of the OMA appear to be rather better (Table 3.8). All antibodies included in this analysis gave strongly positive reactions (3+ to 4+). The overall error rate of antibody detection was 8.5 per 1000 opportunities and there was no trend to improvement. Errors of detection of two weak antibodies (anti-D and anti-P_1) issued in 1976 amounted respectively to 630 and 745 per 1000 opportunities! In Ontario all participating laboratories are now expected to be able to test for irregular antibodies although they are not all expected to be able to identify the antibodies. In 1976 only 44.2 per cent of participants correctly identified a potent anti-D, in 1977 42.4 per cent identified an anti-K and 39.8 per cent identified an anti-c. A weak anti-D issued in 1976 was detected by 26.6 per cent of participants and identified by 23.4 per cent of the participants and a weak anti-P_1 was identified by 13.7 per cent. In the reports of the Royal College of Pathologists of Australia error rates in antibody identification are higher even than those reported in the CAP program but the problems posed have been more difficult and have included uncommon antibodies and also antibody mixtures.[24]

Table 3.8 Error rates for antibody detection (Ontario Medical Association).

Year	Antibody	Error per 1000 Opportunities
1976	D	19.7
1977	K	10.2
	c + E	5.1
1978	D	21.5
	D + Fy^a	0
	Le^a + Le^b	8.0
1979	c + K	4.0
	D	12.2
	k	0
	nl	4.1

Compatibility testing

The incidence of false negative compatibility tests reported in CAP surveys for the period 1973–1977 is given in Table 3.9. The organizers of the CAP program consider that the level of performance is generally satisfactory. There have been several surveys in which the error rates have been clearly unacceptable, but there have usually been mitigating circumstances. For example, an anti-P_1 missed by 41.7 per cent of participants, was active primarily at 12 to 16°C; an anti-S missed by 42.6 per cent of participants was very weak and an anti-Lu^b, missed by 7.5 per cent of participants, reacted with the cells which had been designated as those of the patient.

The CDC has also shown that the error rates in compatibility testing are de-

Table 3.9 Error rates in compatibility tests (College of American Pathologists).

Year	Antibody specificity	Errors per 100 participants
1973	$-P_1$	41.7
	$-e + C$	1.5
	$-K$	1.6
1974	$-E$	6.5
	$-e + Ce$	0.4
	$-e + Ce$	2.6
1975	$-K$	6.9
	$-K$	4.8
	$-I$	0.2
	$-Fy^a + K$	1.6
1976	$-D$	0.1
	$-D$	0.1
	$-S$	42.6
	$-c$	0.3
	$-c$	2.1
	$-K$	1.1
1977	$-c + E$	1.0
	$-Lu^b$	7.5
	$-Lu^b$	2.7
	$-C + D$	0.2
	$-C + D$	0.6

pendent on the nature of the material issued in the surveys. The error rate in compatibility testing reported by the OMA compared favorably to the rates reported by the CAP and the CDC but the experience of the OMA in compatibility testing is limited to a single survey.

The United Kingdom National External Quality Assessment Scheme

In the United Kingdom proficiency testing in blood group serology has been devoted entirely to compatibility testing. This program is supported by the Department of Health and Social Security and was initiated on a national basis in 1979. In each survey five sera are issued, each of which is to be tested by three techniques (saline, albumin and antiglobulin) with each of three cells. The use of the same techniques by every participant facilitates computerization, scoring and comparison of results. The surveys have been accompanied by questionnaires by means of which details of the methodology of antiglobulin testing of each participant have been obtained. This information has been used to establish correlations between performance and technique in antiglobulin testing. Proficiency testing materials are distributed to participants by way of the regional transfusion centres. These centres are the agencies on which hospital blood banks depend for their blood supplies. The participation in this scheme of virtually all blood banks in the UK which undertake compatibility testing has thus been assured.

The overall results of the surveys in the UK in 1979 are given in Table 3.10. Error rates are comparable to those reported by the CAP and CDC. In each of

42 QUALITY CONTROL

Table 3.10 Error rates for compatibility tests (United Kingdom National Scheme).

Survey	Antibody	Total no. of participants	No. of missed incompatibilities	Total no. of participants in error
79–1	K C + D E E	340	9 2 17 75	75(22%)
79–2	Fy^a S K K D	382	11 9 4 4 2	18(4.7%)
79–3	D D S S K	387	0 1 33 38 5	48(12.4%)

the three surveys at least one incompatibility was missed by 4.7 per cent to 22 per cent of participants. Two or more incompatibilities were missed in each survey by 1.8 to 7.0 per cent of participants. All the antibodies issued were readily detectable by conventional techniques and, with the single exception of an anti-E, gave 3 to 4+ reactions by the antiglobulin test. The anti-E was also detectable by the antiglobulin test but gave weaker reactions.

The surveys of antiglobulin techniques revealed first, that there is an extraordinary lack of technical standardization and second, that methodology is currently in a state of flux. In particular, over the three exercises in 1979 the following major changes were observed:
1. An increase in the number of participants using a tube antiglobulin technique from 72.5 per cent to 77.1 per cent.
2. An increase in the number of participants using a low ionic strength antiglobulin technique from 11.4 per cent to 17.7 per cent.
3. A decline in the number of participants using an 'albumin enhanced' antiglobulin technique from 27.5 per cent to 16.5 per cent.

By contrast the finer details of techniques within the tile and tube techniques have shown little change over this period:

1. Cell concentration. The range employed extended from 2 per cent to '100 per cent'. The use of apparently inappropriate concentrations of cells was observed with both tile and tube techniques (Table 3.11). In the tile technique 15.8 per cent of participants used cell concentrations of 5 per cent or less. In the tube technique 17.3 per cent of participants used cell concentrations in excess of 10 per cent including 10 participants who used a 50 per cent cell concentration. A number of participants appeared to have converted from a tile to a tube technique without reducing the cell concentration. Quite apart from the difficulty of reading a tube test at high cell concentration, these participants will have gained no increase in sensitivity through use of a tube technique.

2. Ratio of volume of serum to volume of cell suspension. The ratios employed

Table 3.11 The concentration of cells employed by participants using tile or tube antiglobulin techniques.

% Cells	Tile No.	Tile %	Tube No.	Tube %
0 – 2.5	1	1.3	12	4.8
– 5	11	14.5	148	59.7
– 7.5	1	1.3	12	4.8
– 10	8	10.5	33	13.3
– 20	12	15.8	17	6.9
– 30	11	14.5	13	5.2
– 40			2	0.8
– 50	29	38.2	10	4.0
– 75				
– 100	3	3.9	1	0.4
	76		248	

in the tile and tube techniques were broadly similar and over 80 per cent use ratios of 1/1 to 4/1.

3. *Ratio of volume of serum to volume of cells.* For a given concentration of antibody the amount of antibody bound to cells at equilibrium is dependent on this ratio. Ratios achieved by many using the tube technique were higher than the ratios of those using the tile technique (Table 3.12). This difference was almost entirely due to the use of lower cell concentrations in the tube technique.

4. *Ratio of volume of serum to volume of cell suspension in the low ionic strength technique.* A well known pitfall of the use of low ionic strength techniques is the addition of an excessive volume of serum (i.e. ratio > 1/1) when the cells are suspended in low ionic strength solution. Twenty-five per cent of those who claimed to employ a low ionic strength technique used serum to cell suspension volume ratios in the range 2/1 to 6/1.

5. *Incubation time* The incubation times used with normal ionic strength techniques varied from 15 to more than 120 minutes and the times used with low ionic strength varied from five to 60 minutes.

6. *Number of cell washes.* In the tile technique there was a marked prefer-

Table 3.12 The ratio of volume of serum to volume of cells employed by participants using tile or tube antiglobulin techniques.

Ratio	Tile No.	Tile %	Tube No.	Tube %
0 – 10/1	36	48	23	9.3
– 20	23	30.7	62	2.5
– 30	6	8	26	10.5
– 40	6	8	58	23.4
– 50	3	4	16	6.5
– 60			21	8.5
– 80			21	8.5
– 100	1	1.3	11	4.4
– 150			6	2.4
>150			4	1.6
	75		248	

ence (87 per cent) for four washes whereas in the tube technique 45 per cent considered three washes adequate.

7. *Tube size.* The majority of laboratories employed 75 × 10 mm or 75 × 12 mm tubes. These sizes are necessitated by automated washers. However, smaller tubes were used by 13.7 per cent of participants for the tile technique and by 10.7 per cent for the tube technique.

8. *Wash volume.* A minority of participants (5.7 per cent) used 2 ml or less of saline for each cell wash and 2.1 per cent used volumes of 1 ml or less. Not all of these participants compensated for low wash volumes by increasing the number of washes and the efficiency of cell washing of these participants must have been suspect.

9. *Wash technique.* Manual washing techniques were used by 44 per cent of those using tile technique but by only 14 per cent of those using the tube techniques. This suggests that the purchase of an automated cell washer, in which the tubes can also be spun following the addition of antiglobulin has acted as a considerable spur to convert from a tile to a tube technique.

10. *Manufacturer of antiglobulin reagent.* There are at least 20 different manufacturers from whom polyspecific antiglobulin reagents may be obtained in the United Kingdom. Half of these are of commercial origin and the other half are produced by public bodies, mostly regional transfusion centres. The UK market is, however, dominated by commercial imported reagents and the product of one particular manufacturer is used by 37 per cent of participants for the tile technique and by 48 per cent for the tube technique. It is noteworthy that the manufacturer of this product makes no claim that the reagent is suitable for use with the tile technique.

11. *Volume of antiglobulin reagent used.* In the tube technique 62 per cent used two volumes and 38 per cent used one volume of antiglobulin to one volume of cell suspension. The cost of antiglobulin reagent per test to the former will of course be twice the cost to the latter. Any benefit of the more costly procedure must, therefore, be established.

12. *Centrifugation r/min and RCF.* For the majority these variables are preset by the manufacturers of the automated centrifuges. The three major manufacturers of automated centrifuges have each selected a different RCF for the centrifugation phase which follows the addition of antiglobulin. In consequence the RCF employed varied widely and showed a bimodal disribution with 66 per cent of participants using an RCF in the range 400 to 800 g and 29 per cent using an RCF of 100 to 200 g. The r/min (and RCF) obtained in automated centrifuges should be determined at least monthly by means of an independent instrument such as a tachometer or stroboscope. If it can be assumed that the number of participants who failed to answer specific questions in the questionnaire was the same as the number who did not know the answers then 32 per cent of participants did not know the r/min and 73 per cent did not know the RCF provided by their centrifuges for the final phase of the antiglobulin test. As quality control cannot be applied to a centrifuge in a state of ignorance of the manufacturers' specifications for r/min and RCF it may safely be assumed that the majority of participants in these surveys are applying but rudimentary quality control to their equipment.

13. Centrifugation time. The time that follows the addition of antiglobulin may or may not be pre-set by the manufacturer. As in the case of centrifugation r/min and RCF there was a wide range in use and a bimodal distribution with 57 per cent of participants using 40 to 60 seconds and 33 per cent using 10 to 30 seconds.

14. Reading the results. Results were read macroscopically by 96 per cent of participants for the tile technique and by 76 per cent for the tube technique. Results were read microscopically by 23 per cent of participants for the tile technique. For the tube technique results were routinely read microscopically by 65 per cent of participants and by another 5 per cent on occasions.

Correlation of performance with methodology

While it has been easy to demonstrate apparent deficiencies or aberrations of technique it has been difficult to confirm that any of these factors have contributed in any consistent way to failures of performance. No correlations with performance have been found with such technical 'faults' as the use of inappropriate cell concentration, low serum to cell volume ratio, excess serum volume in low ionic strength techniques or the use of very small wash volumes. Most of these faults would have resulted in only partial loss of sensitivity and the capacity to detect the potent antibodies issued in these surveys was, therefore, little affected. Results obtained with other antibodies covering a wider range of potencies and specificities may prove to be more revealing of the influence of these variables on performance.

Significant effects upon performance have been demonstrated but these depended upon the primary choice of technique rather than on misuse of the selected technique. Effects upon performance are related to the use of:
1. Tile or tube technique.
2. Normal or low ionic strength.
3. 'Albumin enhancement'.

Table 3.13 A comparison of the number and per cent of participants who missed antibodies by the tile or tube antiglobulin test.

	Tile No.	Tile %	Tube No.	Tube %	p =
QC 79-1					
-K	7	9.2	6	2.4	<0.01
-E	22	28.9	22	8.9	<0.001
-E	55	72.4	82	33.1	<0.001
	n = 76		n = 248		
QC 79-2					
-Fy^a	3	3.7	7	2.6	>0.05
-S	3	3.7	6	2.2	>0.05
	n = 82		n = 271		
QC 79-3					
-S	10	14.1	27	9.4	>0.05
-S	7	9.9	31	10.8	>0.05
-K	3	4.2	2	0.7	<0.05
	n = 71		n = 287		

In Table 3.13 the specificities of the antibodies issued are shown together with the number and percentage of participants who missed them by tile or tube antiglobulin technique. On four out of eight possible occasions performance with the tube technique has been significantly better than performance with the tile technique. On no occasion has the tile technique shown a significant advantage. The number and percentage of participants who missed the same antibodies by low or normal ionic strength tube antiglobulin technique are shown in Table 3.14. On two occasions (the same anti-S but with different cells)

Table 3.14 A comparison of the number and per cent of participants who missed antibodies by tube antiglobulin technique using normal (NIS) or low (LIS) ionic strength saline.

	NIS No.	%	LIS No.	%	p =
QC 79–1					
−K	5	2.3	1	3.1	>0.05
−E	19	8.8	3	9.4	>0.05
−E	73	34.0	8	25.0	>0.05
	n = 215		n = 32		
QC 79–2					
−Fy^a	5	2.3	2	3.8	>0.05
−S	6	2.7	0	0	>0.05
	n = 218		n = 52		
QC 79–3					
−S	27	11.8	0	0	<0.01
−S	31	13.5	0	0	<0.01
−K	2	0.9	0	0	>0.05
	n = 229		n = 57		

the use of low ionic strength in the tube technique was of significant advantage and the advantage was gained irrespective of the serum to cell volume ratio used. The effect of the presence or absence of albumin on the number and percentage of participants who missed these antibodies by tube antiglobulin technique is shown in Table 3.15. On three occasions the addition of albumin gave significantly worse results and on no occasion has the use of albumin significantly improved performance.

Standardization of the antiglobulin technique

It is apparent that 35 years after the introduction of the antiglobulin test into routing use[25] there is, in the UK at least, little agreement as to what constitutes a standardized procedure. It might have been hoped that the recent introduction of low ionic strength techniques would have been accompanied by an improvement in standardization but the evidence from the UK surveys is to the contrary. The wide range of variables employed with normal ionic strength techniques has been retained and the introduction of low ionic strength techniques has served merely to introduce a new important variable. The problem is now being compounded by the activities of commercial companies some of whom have devised

Table 3.15 A comparison of the number and per cent of participants who missed antibodies by the tube antiglobulin technique in the presence and absence of added albumin.

	Without albumin		With albumin		p =
	No.	%	No.	%	
QC 79–1					
–K	3	1.7	3	4.1	>0.05
–E	11	6.3	11	14.9	<0.05
–E	52	29.9	30	40.5	>0.05
	n = 174		n = 74		
QC 79–2					
–Fy$_a$	7	3.3	0	0	>0.05
–S	5	2.4	1	1.7	>0.05
	n = 212		n = 60		
QC 79–3					
–S	11	4.8	16	27.6	<0.001
–S	13	5.7	18	31.0	<0.001
–K	1	0.4	1	1.7	>0.05
	n = 229		n = 58		

their own LISS formulae and issued LISS reagents complete with recommended techniques considered appropriate to the new formulae. These commercial products may even contain 'potentiators' such as albumin and the way will soon be clear for the breakdown of what little standardization remains. It is however easier to lament the lack of standardization than to recommend a technique or techniques, the reliability of which has been established in many routine laboratories. It cannot be assumed that techniques which work well in specialist or reference laboratories will prove to be the most reliable in routine laboratories and the very diversity of techniques in use may be a reflection of this.

It is clear from the results of the UK surveys that a number of the incompatibilities that remained undetected would not have been missed if participants had chosen an alternative technique. It is, however, also clear that many incompatibilities were missed by participants who appeared to be using appropriate techniques in the correct manner. Failure to detect the potent antibodies issued in these surveys implies gross loss of sensitivity. It is therefore surprising that the causes of these errors continue to evade identification by the participating laboratories or by external surveillance. The following test and quality control procedures are recommended in the interests of improved standardization and in the hope that standardization may facilitate the identification of the causes of technical errors in antiglobulin testing. For laboratories that cannot reliably detect potent antibodies that are readily demonstrated by conventional techniques, the introduction of a low ionic strength technique would be premature. The use of albumin would appear to be an unnecessary and perhaps even an undesirable complication.

There are many sources of reference available to laboratories which wish to introduce standardized technical procedures for blood group serology.[26–34]

These include recommendations for quality control procedures for reagents and equipment. The evidence obtained from the UK and other national quality assessment schemes suggests that much of this good advice has so far fallen on deaf ears.

RECOMMENDED TECHNIQUES INDIRECT ANTIGLOBULIN TEST

A. Tile technique, normal ionic strength
1. Prepare a 20 per cent suspension of washed red cells.
2. Add four volumes of serum to one volume of cell suspension in a 75 × 10 mm or 75 × 12 mm tube and mix well.
3. Incubate at 37°C for 60 min.
4. Wash cells four times leaving a 30 per cent cell suspension.
5. Add one volume of antiglobulin reagent to one volume of 30 per cent cell suspension on an opaque glass tile.
6. Mix well.
7. Read results after 5 min over a diffuse light.

B. Tube technique, normal ionic strength
1. Prepare a 3 per cent suspension of washed red cells.
2. Add two volumes of serum to one volume of cell suspension in a 75 × 10 mm or 75 × 12 mm tube and mix well.
3. Incubate at 37°C for 60 min.
4. Wash the cells three times.
5. Add two volumes of antiglobulin reagent and mix well.
6. Centrifuge the tube immediately for 60s at 1200 r/min (130 g) or for 15 s at 3600 r/min (1200 g) or at a suitable intermediate r/min (g) and time in an automated system.
7. Gently shake the tube and observe macroscopically for agglutination over a white background. Check the negatives microscopically.

C. Tube technique, low ionic strength
1. Prepare a 3 per cent suspension of washed red cells suspended in low ionic strength solution* (LISS). Wash cells twice in isotonic saline, once in LISS and resuspend cells to 3 per cent in LISS.
2. Add one volume[†] of serum to one volume[†] of cell suspension in a 75 × 10 mm or 75 × 12 mm tube and mix well.
3. Incubate at 37°C for 15 min.
4. Wash the cells three times with isotonic saline.
5. Add two volumes of antiglobulin reagent and mix well.
6. Centrifuge the tube immediately for 60 s at 1200 r/min (130 g) or for 15 s at

---

* LISS formula: see Mollison P L 1979, Blood transfusion in clinical medicine, 6th edn. Blackwell, Oxford, Appendix 11, p 739.
[†] The use of an automatic pipette is recommended, one volume = 50 μl, see Moore H C, Mollison P L 1976 Transfusion. (Philad.) 16: 291.

3600 r/min (1200 g) or at a suitable intermediate r/min (g) and time in an automated system.
7. Gently shake the tube and observe macroscopically for agglutination over a white background. Check the negatives microscopically.

Quality control, indirect antiglobulin test
Control is required of all aspects of the antiglobulin test including the technique, the reagents, the equipment and the performer.
1. Control of the technique, the reagents and the performer can be achieved by setting up a compatibility test with a weak anti-D with each batch of compatibility tests undertaken.
2. Control is also required of the functions of automated cell washers. This can be achieved by the addition of strongly sensitized cells to *each* negative compatibility test. This procedure acts not only as a control of the adequacy of cell washing of each test sample and of the addition of antiglobulin to each test sample but also of the reagent and of the final phases of the test.

RECOMMENDED TECHNIQUES — DIRECT ANTIGLOBULIN TEST

A. Tile technique
1. Prepare a 30 per cent cell suspension of four times washed cells.
2. Add one volume of antiglobulin reagent to one volume of 30 per cent cell suspension on an opal glass tile.
3. Mix well.
4. Read results after 5 min over a diffuse light.

B. Tube technique
1. Prepare a 3 per cent cell suspension of four times washed cells.
2. Add two volumes of antiglobulin reagent to one volume of 3 per cent cells in a 75 × 10 mm or 75 × 12 mm tube and mix well.
3. Centrifuge the tube immediately for 60 s at 1200 r/min (130 g) or for 15 s at 3600 r/min (120 g) or at a suitable intermediate r/min (g) and time in an automated system.
4. Gently shake the tube and observe macroscopically for agglutination over a white background. Check the negatives microspically.

REFERENCES

1. Myhre B A 1974 Quality Control in blood banking. Wiley, New York, ch 1, p 2
2. Harrison G E 1976 Equipment evaluation and maintenance. In: Myhre B A (ed) A seminar on performance evaluation. Gunthrop-Warren Printing Company, Chicago, p 121–133.
3. Grindon A J, Eska P L 1977 Error rate, precision and accuracy in immunohaematology. Transfusion 17: 425–430
4. Greendyke R M, Wormer J L, Banzhaf M S 1978 Quality assurance in the blood bank. American Journal of Clinical Pathology 71: 286–290
5. Schmidt P J, Kevy S V 1963 Sources of error in a hospital blood bank. Transfusion 3: 198–201

6. Kwa S B, Ariff K B Md 1966 Blood banking errors — a two year prospective study. Singapore Medical Journal 7: 178–184
7. Taswell H F, Smith A M, Sweatt M A, Pfaff K J 1974 Quality Control in the blood bank — a new approach. American Journal of Clinical Pathology 62: 491–495
8. Taswell H F 1976 Error production and its control. In: Myhre B A (ed) A seminar on performance evaluation, Gunthrop-Warren Printing Company, Chicago, p 115–120
9. Taswell H F, Sonnenberg C L 1979 Blood bank errors: a new functional classification. Transfusion 19: 652–653
10. Koepke J A, Eilers R J 1967 A survey of clinical laboratory immunohematology performance. Transfusion: 7 316–318
11. Koepke J A 1970 Immunohematology proficiency testing, 1966–1969. American Journal of Clinical Pathology 54 (supplement): 508–511
12. Myhre B A, Koepke J A 1975 The College of American Pathologists comprehensive blood bank survey program, 1973. American Journal of Clinical Pathology 63 (supplement): 995–1001
13. Myhre B A, Koepke J A, Polesky H 1976 The comprehensive blood bank survey program of the College of American Pathologists, 1974. American Journal of Clinical Pathology 66 (supplement): 248–254
14. Myhre B A, Koepke J A, Polesky H F, Walker R, Van Schoonhoven P 1977 The CAP blood bank comprehensive survey program — 1975. American Journal of Clinical Pathology 68 (supplement): 175–179
15. Myhre B A, Koepke J A, Polesky H F, Van Schoonhoven P, Walker R 1978 The comprehensive blood bank survey program of the College of American Pathologists, 1976. American Journal of Clinical Pathology 70 (supplement): 548–553
16. Myhre B A, Mullen S, Polesky H F, Van Schoonhoven P, Walker R 1979 The comprehensive blood bank survey program of the College of American Pathologists — 1977. American Journal of Clinical Pathology 72 (supplement): 352–357
17. Weiner A S 1976 Letter to the Editor. American Journal of Clinical Pathology 65: 254.
18. Walker R H 1976 Proficiency testing — a facet of the total quality assurance program. In: Myhre B A (ed) A seminar on performance evaluation, Gunthrop-Warren Printing Company, Chicago, p 135–145
19. Code of Federal Regulations 1978 US Government Printing Office, Washington, p 143–151
20. Myhre B A, Koepke J A 1976 Letter to the Editor. American Journal of Clinical Pathology 65: 254–256
21. Proficiency Testing Summary Analyses, Immunohematology 1977 I–IV, 1978 I–IV and 1979 I–III US Department of Health, Education and Welfare, Center for Disease Control
22. Pinkerton P H, Wood D E, Burnie K L, Carstairs K C, Croucher B E E, Ezer S et al 1979 Proficiency testing in immunohaemtology in Ontario, Canada, 1975–1977. American Journal of Clinical Pathology 72: 559–563
23. Pinkerton P H, Wood D E, Burnie K L, Carstairs K C, Croucher B E E, Ezer S et al 1980 Proficiency testing in immunohaematology in Ontario, Canada, 1977–1979. Clinical and Laboratory Haematology 3:155–164
24. Reports of Serological Surveys 1975, 1976, 1977 and 1978, Royal College of Pathologists of Australia
25. Coombes R R A, Mourant A E, Race R R 1945 A new test for the detection of weak and 'incomplete' Rh agglutinins. British Journal of Experimental Pathology 26: 255–266.
26. Mollison P L 1979 Blood Transfusion in clinical medicine, 6th edn. Blackwell, Oxford
27. Miller W V (ed) 1977 Technical manual of the American Association of Blood Banks, 7th edn. Lippincott, Philadelphia
28. Moore B P L (ed) 1980 Serological and immunological methods of the Canadian Red Cross Transfusion Service, 8th edn. The Canadian Red Cross Transfusion Service, 8th edn. The Canadian Red Cross Society, Toronto.
29. Considerations in the selection of reagents, a technical workshop 1979. American Association of Blood Banks, Washington
30. Guy L R, Neitzer G M, Klein R E 1977 Quality Control — how much is enough? Transfusion 17: 183–194
31. Wilson M J 1976 Blood bank quality assurance, Blood group immunology. Dade Division, American Hospital Supply Corporation, Miami, p 148–165
32. Issitt P D, Issit C H 1975 Applied blood group serology. Spectra Biologicals Division of Becton, Dickenson
33. Boorman K E, Dodd B E, Lincoln P J 1977 Blood group serology. Theory, techniques, practical applications, 5th edn. Churchill Livingstone, Edinburgh
34. Moore B P L (ed) 1978 International Society of Blood Transfusion Guide 3. Quality control in the blood transfusion laboratory. International Society of Blood Transfusion, Paris.

4
Standardization of Coagulation Tests and Assays

T. W. Barrowcliffe

INTRODUCTION

Attempts to measure the main factors participating in coagulation have been made since their discovery early in the century, but it is only in the last 25 years that reliable specific assays have been developed for most of the clotting factors. The one-stage prothrombin time introduced by Quick[1] was based on the simple principle which is used in many of the more sophisticated tests, namely that of providing an excess or standard amount of all substances necessary for coagulation except the one being measured. The aim of standardization of coagulation tests and assays is to provide a uniform and reproducible system of measurement and this can be seen at three different levels. First, within any one laboratory the results must be consistent over a period of time. The second level of standardization relates results in one laboratory to those in others, the aim being to achieve similarity, if not complete identity, of results. This is normally done at regional or national level. 'Proficiency assessment', as its name implies, is an attempt to monitor performance of laboratories. In these exercises, all laboratories use their own techniques, and so a picture is built up of the 'state of the art'. 'External quality control', however, implies an additional degree of surveillance, in the form of a recommended assay technique for different laboratories to follow, or sometimes the supply of reagents to many different laboratories. When a proficiency assessment scheme shows an unacceptable degree of heterogeneity between laboratories then external quality control may be applied to improve the situation; this is the case, for instance, with the British system for control of oral anticoagulant therapy as described by Thomson.[2] The standardization of reagents and techniques, however, should never precede a thorough investigation into the advantages and disadvantages of the various systems currently in use.

The third, and in many ways most difficult level of standardization, is at the international level. Coagulation techniques and reagents used in different countries are often widely different. Also quality control schemes which are successful in one country are not always applicable to others. Complete standardization of coagulation techniques in different countries is probably not attainable, nor should it be regarded as a desirable end, provided each country can standardize its own methodology satisfactorily. Two international symposia have recently been devoted to this topic[3,4] and the World Health Organization (WHO) has an Expert Committee on Biological Standardization whose reports are published in the WHO Technical Report Series.

In the UK, the two bodies involved in standardization are the National Reference Laboratory for Anticoagulant Reagents and Control (NRLARC), Manchester, and the National Institute for Biological Standards and Control (NIBSC), London. NRLARC was primarily involved in establishing the British system for anticoagulant control, involving widespread proficiency testing of the prothrombin time and national supply of standardized thromboplastin reagents. Its activities have recently been extended to include national proficiency testing of the partial thromboplastin time, and assays of fibrinogen and Factor VIII. NIBSC is a WHO Laboratory for biological standards, and supplies reference standards for several clotting factors; it does not supply routine reagents and is not involved in proficiency testing. A similar situation applies in the USA, where the College of American Pathologists runs large-scale proficiency testing trials, and reference standards are supplied by the Bureau of Biologics. The systems of standardization developed in the UK, USA and other countries have recently been reviewed by Poller.[5]

In this Chapter, progress towards standardization of the main types of clotting test and assay will be reviewed, with particular emphasis on the extent to which national and international agreement has been reached.

COLLECTION OF BLOOD

It is important to ensure first that all specimens are collected in a uniform manner by a method which does not interfere with the subsequent test results. Since virtually all clotting tests are carried out on citrated plasma, a number of manipulations are involved in preparation of the sample, and there are several important points to consider.

Blood/anticoagulant ratio

It has been general practice to adopt a ratio of 9 parts blood to 1 part anticoagulant. This ratio must be adhered to as closely as possible. For patients whose hematocrit is significantly different from 0.450 the ratio should be adjusted to give a constant citrate/plasma ratio.[6] Attempts have been made to use dried citrate but no satisfactory dried citrate tubes are yet available.[7]

Citrate concentration

Several different concentrations of citrate are in common use in the range 0.09 M to 0.15 M. Concentrations above 0.11 M are hypertonic and may induce a small prolongation of the prothrombin time.[6] A concentration of 3.8 per cent w/v is widely used: When trisodium citrate, 5½ H_2O is used this is 0.106 M but if the *dihydrate* salt is used at the same concentration this will give a 0.129 M solution; this is unnecessarily high, and its use should be discontinued. The concentration of the dihydrate required to give 0.106 M is 3.13 per cent, and this is generally rounded up to 3.2 per cent, giving 0.109 M which is recommended for prothrombin times.[8]

Use of buffers

The pH of trisodium citrate anticoagulant solution is around 8.6, and plasma tends to become alkaline on storage due to loss of CO_2. This can be minimized by incorporation of a buffer such as HEPES (N-2 hydroxyethylpiperazine N-2-ethanesulphonic acid) at a concentration of 0.05 M in plasma. This will keep the pH stable and the prothrombin time reproducible for up to eight hours after reconstitution of freeze-dried samples.[9] It also minimizes the loss of Factor VIII on freezing and freeze-drying,[10] and British Standard plasmas for Factor VIII are now prepared with addition of buffer after the first centrifugation.[11]

Centrifugation

Most clotting tests are carried out on platelet-poor plasma, and the technique of centrifugation is a potential source of variation. The main variable to be controlled is the time between collecting blood and starting centrifugation. This should be as short as possible. If whole blood is left standing, platelets may release components which have an effect on subsequent clotting tests. The assessment of heparin, in particular, can be seriously affected by release of the antiheparin protein platelet factor 4 (PF4). Figure 4.1 shows that significant losses of heparin activity may occur after 1 hour, and when centrifugation is delayed for three hours, about 25 per cent of the original activity is neutralized.

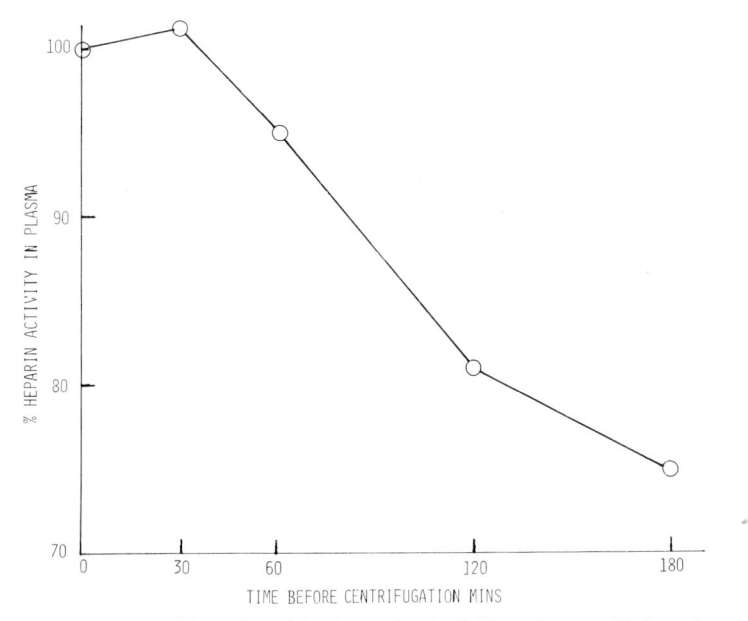

Fig. 4.1 The progressive loss of heparin activity in whole blood. Heparin was added to whole blood to give a plasma concentration of approximately 0.3 iu/ml. Samples of blood were left at room temperature for various intervals before centrifugation, and the heparin concentration measured by three methods (anti-Xa, APTT and thrombin time).

STANDARDIZATION OF SCREENING TESTS

1. THE PROTHROMBIN TIME

The prothrombin time was introduced by Quick in 1935,[1] and it might be thought that in the 45 years since then some measure of agreement would have been reached on the method and its interpretation. That this is not so is a tribute to the coagulationists' ingenuity, in introducing modifications and variations to this most simple of coagulation tests.

The prothrombin time and oral anticoagulants

When Quick introduced the test, the only substances thought to be necessary for thrombin formation were prothrombin, tissue thromboplastin and calcium. It is now known that Factors V, VII and X are also required for optimal activation of prothrombin via the extrinsic (tissue-mediated) pathway, and that the prothrombin time is more sensitive to changes in concentration of these factors than to prothrombin (Factor II) concentration.

Factors II, VII and X are three of the four clotting factors which require vitamin K for their biosynthesis; the fourth is Factor IX, which is involved in the intrinsic pathway of prothrombin activation. Oral anticoagulants of the coumarin type act by inhibition of vitamin K and cause a reduction in concentration of these four factors. Vitamin K is involved in carboxylation of terminal glutamic acid residues in these proteins, and the new amino acids produced, γ-carboxyglutamic acid, are necessary for binding the molecules to calcium and to phospholipid.[12] Under the influence of oral anticoagulants, abnormal molecules of Factors II, VII, IX and X, lacking the extra carboxyl group on their glutamic acid residues, are produced. These proteins were first described by Hemker and colleagues[13,14] and termed PIVKAs (Protein Induced by Vitamin K Absence or Antagonism); more recently, it has been recommended that they be designated 'acarboxy' forms.[15] These abnormal proteins must be taken into consideration when measuring the prothrombin time on samples from patients receiving oral anticoagulants.

Under oral anticoagulant therapy, concentrations of Factors II, VII, IX and X fall to approximately the same degree, though at different rates because of their different plasma half-lives. The prothrombin time is sensitive to three of these factors and is the ideal test for monitoring therapy. The aim of treatment is to achieve a level of anticoagulation sufficient to prevent thrombosis but insufficient to cause hemorrhage. Since dose requirements vary enormously between different individuals, laboratory control is essential, and a therapeutic range can only be defined in terms of results of prothrombin time tests. Efforts at standardization of the prothrombin time have therefore been directed largely towards development of an agreed therapeutic range for oral anticoagulant therapy.

Technical variables and the need for standardization

The original method used oxalated plasma and thromboplastin prepared from rabbit brians.[1] Since then, citrate has largely replaced oxalate as an anticoagulant, and the chief source of variation has been the introduction of various types of thromboplastin reagents. It was soon pointed out[16] that different thromboplastins may give different results. Table 4.1 shows the mean prothrombin times of 12 plasmas from coumarin-treated patients, expressed as ratios to the prothrombin time of normal plasma, with the most commonly used reagents. They cover a twofold range. The main reason for these differences is the species specificity

Table 4.1 Mean prothrombin time ratios of twelve coumarin-treated patients using a variety of commercial thromboplastin reagents and the British Comparative Thromboplastin. (Data reproduced with kind permission from Thomson.[2])

Thromboplastin	Mean ratio
British Comparative Thromboplastin	2.96
Thrombotest	2.47
Thromborel	1.91
Diagen (phenolized)	1.87
Simplastin A	1.83
Diagen (freeze-dried)	1.74
Ortho	1.63
Dade thromboplastin 'C'	1.61
Boehringer	1.57
Hyland	1.55
Simplastin	1.52
Dade activated (liquid)	1.48
Dade (freeze-dried)	1.47

involved in the interaction between tissue factor, a phospholipid/lipoprotein complex, and the human clotting factors, especially VII and X. A variety of tissues from several species have been used as thromboplastin reagents, and it is well established that human brain extracts are most sensitive, and rabbit brain reagents among the least sensitive. Some manufacturers have also added bovine Factor V, fibrinogen and phospholipid to their reagents. However, an unmodified human brain extract remains the most sensitive reagent.

The other main aspect of the prothrombin time which has changed since Quick's original test was described is the method of measuring the clotting time. Automated instruments are being increasingly used, accounting for more than 94 per cent of laboratories in the USA.[17] In the UK, automation is, as yet, much less widespread, with 70 per cent of laboratories still using a manual technique in 1978.[18]

With all these differences it is not surprising that confusion has developed in the definition of the optimal therapeutic range of oral anticoagulants.[19] In addition to the reagent and instrument differences already mentioned, there have also been three methods of expressing the results:

1. Prothrombin index, i.e. $\frac{\text{normal prothrombin time}}{\text{patient's prothrombin time}} \times 100$
2. Prothrombin activity, expressed as a percentage from a dilution curve obtained with normal plasma
3. Prothrombin ratio, i.e.
$$\frac{\text{patient's prothrombin time (s)}}{\text{normal prothrombin time (s)}}$$

Prothrombin index is now hardly used. The percentage activity from a dilution curve was formerly the most popular, but it is now recognized that the percentage activity measured will still be dependent on the reagent used and, since the discovery of the PIVKA proteins, that dilutions of normal plasma cannot substitute for coumarin plasma. In addition, the errors of measurement using a dilution curve are greater than with the ratio method, and in recent years there has been a general trend towards adoption of the ratio method, originally suggested by Biggs in 1965.[20]

The technical differences in measuring prothrombin time are reflected in reported differences in therapeutic ranges. In a French survey 30 per cent activity was considered in some centres to represent the optimum lower limit while in others it represented the safe upper limit.[21] A similar state of affairs was found at an international level.[22] Clearly this situation can only be improved by either eliminating the differences between test systems, or finding some means of relating results obtained in one system to those with another. The following sections describe various different approaches to this problem.

The British system for anticoagulant control

The British system has developed from the introduction of a well characterized, sensitive human brain thromboplastin reagent by Dr L. Poller and Dr J. M. Thomson at the Withington Hospital, Manchester. When this Manchester Comparative Reagent (MCR), was made available its use soon spread to over half the hospitals in the UK. Results from hospitals using different thromboplastins were related to the others by designating batches of MCR as reference reagents, the 'British Comparative Thromboplastin (BCT)', against which other thromboplastins could be compared. The method of calibrating one thromboplastin against a reference preparation[23] is shown in Figure 4.2. The prothrombin times of several plasmas from patients and normal subjects are measured with both reagents. The results (expressed as ratios relative to normal plasma) for the test reagent are plotted against those for the reference reagent, and a 'best fit' line

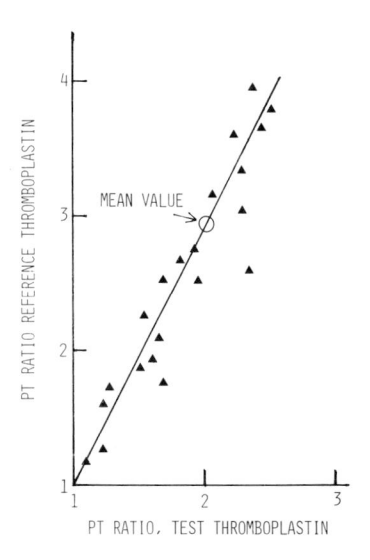

Fig. 4.2 Comparison of two thromboplastins, using prothrombin time ratios obtained from 20 patients' samples with each reagent. The mean value of the 20 ratios is calculated for each thromboplastin and the line joining this point to the origin is the 'mean values line' (see text p. 61). Any PT ratio obtained with the test thromboplastin can be converted to that with the reference thromboplastin, as shown on the graph.

through the points drawn by eye. Any prothrombin time ratio measured with the test reagent can then be converted to that which would be obtained with the reference reagent by interpolation from the graph, or by calculation from the slope of the line.

Samples of BCT were sent to all hospitals not using the Manchester reagent, so that each hospital could calibrate its local reagent, whether home-produced or commercial, against BCT. Hospitals could then report the ratio which they would have been obtained using the Manchester Reagent; this 'British Corrected Ratio' (BCR) has provided a common scale for prothrombin time measurement in the UK. Although BCT was used by many hospitals when first introduced, the majority (>90 per cent) have since switched to the routine reagent MCR. The measures taken to ensure the quality and consistency of large-scale production batches are described in detail by Poller and Ingram[24] and reviewed by Thomson.[2] Batches are checked against a master reference thromboplastin, using both freeze-dried and fresh coumarin plasmas. In addition, an independent monitoring scheme was set up to calibrate successive batches of BCT, involving 12 hospitals.

Other aspects of the British system are the introduction of a standardized technique for prothrombin time measurement (described in the ACP Broadsheet No. 71, and reproduced in Appendix I p. 77) and the establishment of a proficiency assessment scheme. In this scheme,[25] samples of the same freeze dried coumarin plasmas are sent to over 400 centres, who are asked to measure prothrombin times using BCT and the recommended technique. Since all results should theoretically be identical, the percentage deviation from the mean prothrombin ratio gives an indication of interlaboratory variation. Since the introduction of the scheme, there has been a continuous improvement in the overall performance of participants.[26] A similar system to that in the UK has developed in Holland, with most laboratories using the same reagent, Thrombotest. Successive batches of reagent are carefully calibrated, using a simplified version[27] of the calibration procedure described in Figure 4.2. As in the UK, there is a proficiency assessment scheme.[28]

In most countries, however, many different thromboplastin reagents continue to be used, although some countries have established national reference reagents along the lines of the BCT. In Australia, for example, a national human brain thromboplastin reagent which has been calibrated against BCT is available but in 1978 there were still major differences in the therapeutic ranges used in clinical practice.[29]

Reference plasmas
In the USA the establishment of a national standard reagent has been impracticable for geographical and other reasons. An alternative approach to standardization has been developed using reference plasmas[30] and this is based on the therapeutic range in terms of percentages of clotting factors. Large batches of plasma, artificially depleted of the vitamin K dependent clotting factors, are prepared and their prothrombin times measured with all the different thromboplastins currently in use.[31] If the therapeutic range is then defined in terms of the content of a particular factor, the prothrombin times corresponding to this

Table 4.2 Therapeutic ranges for the control of oral anticoagulant therapy with various commercial thromboplastins, representing a reduction of the Factor VII content to 10 to 20% of normal (Data reproduced with kind permission of Dr. J.B. Miale[31]).

Thromboplastin	Therapeutic range (s)
British Comparative	30–53
Hyland (dried)	22–36
Simplastin	22–36
Fibroplastin	22–30
Simplastin A	21–30
Thrombotime	24–30
Ortho	15–30
Dade (dried)	17–26
Dade (activated)	15–21

range can then be easily determined for the different reagents. The concept is illustrated for Factor VII in Figure 4.3, and the therapeutic ranges obtained for the different reagents are shown in Table 4.2.

There are two major drawbacks to the use of reference plasmas as the primary system of standardization. Firstly, even in plasmas collect carefully and freeze-dried by methods used to preserve international biological reference materials, the vitamin K dependent factors were relatively unstable.[32,33] When stored at +4°C, predicted losses over 10 years were around 50 per cent for Factor X, up to 18 per cent for Factor VII, and up to 30 per cent for Factor II. Even at −20°C, up to 8 per cent of the original Factor X activity could be lost after 10 years. A second problem arises from the differences which exist between artificially depleted freeze-dried plasmas and fresh plasmas from coumarin treated patients.[34] Because of the absence of PIVKAs in the artificially produced plasmas, comparative results with different thromboplastin reagents may differ from

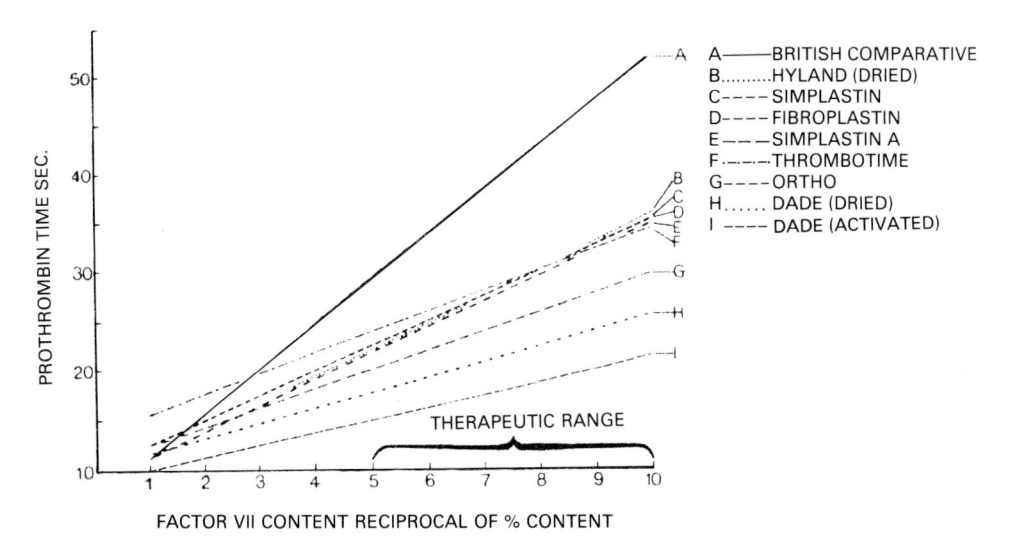

Fig. 4.3 Prothrombin times with nine thromboplastins plotted against reciprocal of percentage Factor VII concentration in a reference plasma. (Data reproduced with the kind permission of Dr J.B. Miale[31])

those obtained on fresh coumarin plasmas. Even freeze-dried plasma from oral anticoagulant patients is not identical to fresh plasma, because of the activation of Factor VII which occurs on lyophilization. The concentration of Factors VII and X measured may also vary with the thromboplastin reagent used.[34] In spite of these drawbacks, reference plasmas can be used in calibration of thromboplastins, in proficiency assessment schemes, and in internal quality control.[27]

The benchmark system
There are 90 possible combinations of instrument and thromboplastin in the USA, and in a survey carried out by the College of American Pathologists[35] 38 of these were in use. In an attempt to interrelate these various systems, one particular combination of thromboplastin and reagent was chosen as a 'benchmark' system, against which results using other systems could be compared. In the CAP proficiency assessment surveys samples of the same freeze-dried plasma are sent out to over 4000 participating laboratories. The prothrombin times on a particular batch of plasma are calculated as ratios to that obtained with the benchmark system. Comparisons with the benchmark reagent and different instruments give a series of 'method ratios', whilst comparisons of different thromboplastins with the benchmark instrument give a series of 'thromboplastin ratios'. This is illustrated for a normal pooled plasma in Table 4.3. The prothrombin time for any reagent/instrument combination can then be calculated as follows:

Calculated PT = benchmark PT × method ratio × thromboplastin ratio

For example, for laboratories using the Electra method with thromboplastin No. 5,

the calculated PT = 20.11 × 0.92 × 0.97 = 17.95 s

The actual mean value obtained by a group of 72 laboratories using this combination was 18.24 seconds, a difference of 1.6 per cent from the calculated value. In a series of such calculations, the mean difference of the actual values from the calculated ones was 2.25 per cent, although differences of up to 8.6 per cent were found with some reagent/instrument combinations. These calcula-

Table 4.3 Calculation of prothrombin time ratios using the benchmark system* (Koepke et al., 1977)[†35]

Thromboplastin	Tilt tube	Fibrometer	Methods Electra	Coagulyzer	BioData
1	17.48	17.38 (0.86)	16.58	16.27	—
2	16.97	16.70 (0.83)	—	—	—
3	20.51 (1.02)	20.11 (1.00)	18.47 (0.92)	17.30 (0.86)	17.42 (0.87)
4	19.52	18.48 (0.92)	—	—	—
5	19.75	19.46 (0.97)	18.24	16.56	17.09
7	18.45	18.01 (0.90)	16.06	15.27	15.92
8	—	18.00 (0.90)	—	—	—
9	18.87	17.97 (0.89)	—	—	—

* The 'benchmark' system is the fibrometer with thromboplastin No. 3.
† Gratitude is expressed to Dr J A Koepke for permission to reproduce some of his original data in Table 4.3.

tions were performed on normal plasma only, and the errors on artificially depleted plasmas are likely to be higher, for reasons already discussed. Although the system will probably be helpful in comparisons of different instruments, it seems unlikely to resolve the basic problem of defining the therapeutic range with different thromboplastin reagents.

Reference thromboplastins
If one preparation were established as a reference material of proven stability this could serve as a standard for calibrating all other reagents. In 1967, a batch of human brain reagent combined with bovine Factor V and fibrinogen became available as a potential standard. This material, coded NIBSC 67/40, was compared to a similarly ampouled bovine reagent, 68/434.[36] Results from the three participating laboratories were very similar, indicating that comparison of thromboplastins could be carried out on a reproducible basis by different laboratories. Accelerated degradation studies on reagent 67/40 indicated some lengthening of clotting times after storage for two years at $+20°C$, but the ratio of abnormal to normal plasma remained the same and, at $-20°C$, the normal storage temperature, the reagent was predicted to be very stable. Denson[37] showed how reagent 67/40 could be used to achieve national and international standardization. A more extensive collaborative study in which four freeze-dried thromboplastins (one human, one bovine and two rabbit) were compared to 67/40, using freeze-dried plasmas showed that results were similar in the four participating laboratories,[38] but the comparison of thromboplastins from the same species was more precise than that between reagents from different species. Results with the freeze-dried patients' plasmas were similar to those with fresh plasmas, but the artificial plasmas gave different results, indicating that they were unsuitable for thromboplastin calibration. It has been suggested that the four thromboplastin reagents studied be used as secondary reference standards for calibrating reagents of similar species and type, their sensitivity having been established by comparison with the proposed standard, 67/40.

Towards international standardization
In 1974 a joint Expert Panel set up by the International Committee on Thrombosis and Hemostasis (ICTH) and the International Committee for Standardization in Hematology (ICSH) initiated a study, with the overall aim of establishing a common scale for measurement of the prothrombin time with different thromboplastins.

It involved 199 laboratories, nine commercial thromboplastins, the British Comparative Thromboplastin (BCT) and four of the NIBSC proposed reference thromboplastins.

The results of the study[39] confirmed what had been previously found in smaller studies,[36,38] namely that different thromboplastins could be validly compared against each other, and against a common reference thromboplastin, using the method of Biggs and Denson.[23] The proposed reference thromboplastin, NIBSC 67/40, was not included in the study but all reagents in the study were compared to the NIBSC rabbit thromboplastin, 70/178, whose sensitivity relative to

Table 4.4 Calibration constants of thromboplastins (Data from ICTH/ICSH study).

Reagent	Calibration constant
Simplastin A	0.81
Thrombotest	1.01
BCT	1.01
Thromborel	0.77
Simplastin	0.34
Ortho	0.36
Dade	0.39
Merieux	0.42
Stago	0.48
Lyoplastin	0.34
NIBSC 68/434	1.02
NIBSC 69/223	0.84
NIBSC 70/115	1.06

Calibrated ratio (CR) is determined from observed ratio (PTR$_{obs}$) and calibration constant (CC) as follows:

$$CR = 1 + \left(\frac{PTR_{obs} - 1}{CC}\right)$$

For example, for Simplastin, a ratio of 1.5 corresponds to

$$1 + \left(\frac{1.5 - 1}{0.34}\right) = 2.47 \text{ on the calibrated scale}$$

67/40 was known.[38] Thus the slopes of all reagents plotted against 67/40 could be calculated; these slopes are the calibration constants of the thromboplastins (Table 4.4). and can be used to convert the observed prothrombin time ratio with any known reagent to a common 'calibrated scale', either graphically, as shown in Figure 4.2, or from the formula given at the foot of Table 4.4.

One of the major difficulties encountered during the study was deciding the method to be used for plotting the graph of prothrombin time ratios obtained with two thromboplastins. Two methods which have been used are the best fit by eye, and calculation of the regression line. A third method, which was eventually used to calculate the calibration constants, is to draw a straight line from the origin (1, 1) to the point of intersection of the mean ratios for each thromboplastin, the so-called 'mean values' line (Fig. 4.2). One of the difficulties with this method is that the line must pass through the origin, even though this is not always the case in reality. An alternative to the basic method of plotting prothrombin time ratios has been suggested in which the prothrombin times (seconds) for both normal and patients' plasmas are plotted for the two thromboplastins, each on a log scale.[40] The line can be fitted by eye, as with the previous method, or by orthogonal regression analysis. If prothrombin time ratios are still preferred these are related to each other by a simple formula in which the value of the slope is all that is required to convert ratios with any reagent to the ratio which would be obtained with the reference thromboplastin. This method is described in Appendix III, p. 79.

This alternative method has a number of advantages, among which are that it takes into account the error involved in measuring the normal prothrombin time.

The method is being tested in a European collaborative study and preliminary indications are that the method provides a reproducible and accurate method of comparing thromboplastins.

WHO recommendations

THE WHO Expert Committee on Biological Standardization has made a series of recommendations on prothrombin time standardization. The basis of the WHO system is the establishment of an international scale for measurement of prothrombin time ratios, called the international calibrated ratio scale. To be successful, the system requires the cooperation of WHO to establishing and distribute reference thromboplastins, the manufacturers of thromboplastins to calibrate their reagents, and hematologists to report their results in international calibrated ratios (ICRs).

International reference thromboplastins

As a result of the ICSH/ICTH study, three of the NIBSC thromboplastins were designated international reference preparations (IRPs), with defined international calibration constants. These are: 67/40 (human brain), 70/178 (rabbit) and 68/434 (bovine) and are available on request from the Division of Blood Products, NIBSC. Because of reduced stocks and the age of the preparations, all are likely to be replaced within the next few years and the new international reference preparations will be held and distributed by the laboratory of the Dutch Thrombosis Service, University Hospital, Leiden.

Calibration of reagents

It is hoped that all manufacturers will calibrate their reagents against the appropriate IRP in a two-tier process. A working reference preparation should be established by each manufacturer, and this reagent carefully calibrated against the appropriate IRP, using fresh normal and patients' plasma as previously described. The working reference preparation can then be used to calibrate successive batches of reagent, using fresh, frozen, or freeze-dried plasmas from normals and patients. The calibration constants should be determined to an accuracy of at least 2 per cent (expressed as a coefficient of variation, CV) for the working reference preparation and 3 per cent for each batch.

Calculation of international calibrated ratios (ICR)

The establishment of international reference thromboplastins, and the calibration of reagents against these, could eventually lead to the adoption of a common system of measurement, the ICR. Ultimately, it is hoped that all laboratories will report results not as observed PTs or PT ratios but as ICRs, using the following formula:

$$ICR = 1 + \frac{PTR_{obs} - 1}{ICC}$$

where PTR_{obs} = observed prothrombin ratio
ICC = International Calibration Constant

An example of such a calculation is shown at the foot of Table 4.4.

STANDARDIZATION OF SCREENING TESTS

II: THE PARTIAL THROMBOPLASTIN TIME (PTT)

Principles of the test

When plasma is recalcified in the absence of tissue factor, prothrombin activation takes place via the intrinsic system, involving Factors XII, XI, IX, VIII, X and V. In the absence of platelets, recalcification of plasma results in inefficient prothrombin conversion and long, poorly reproducible clotting times. Platelet-rich plasma is difficult to prepare reproducibly. It cannot be used reliably to monitor deficiencies of the intrinsic clotting factors since it will also be sensitive to platelet abnormalities. In an attempt to overcome these problems, the partial thromboplastin time (PTT) was developed, in which platelets were replaced by an artificially produced phospholipid reagent.[41] The clot-promoting activity provided by platelets is a phospholipid mixture generally known as platelet Factor 3. A crude phospholipid mixture, prepared by organic solvent extraction of brain and known as cephalin[42] is used as a substitute for platelets in the PTT.

To minimize PTT variation due to surface contact [43] kaolin was added to provide reproducible surface activation;[44] this also had the effect of shortening the clotting times. Surface activation does not require calcium, and therefore plasma is incubated with kaolin for a specified time before addition of $CaCl_2$. The phospholipid may be added either at the beginning or end of the activation period. The activated PTT (APTT) has largely replaced the original non-activated PTT (NAPTT) as an overall test of the intrinsic system. The use of different reagents and techniques gives rise to the same problem of standardizing the therapeutic range as for the prothrombin time.

Technical variables and their influence on test results

The majority of laboratories use one of the large variety of commercially available APTT reagents which may differ widely in their sensitivity to Factor VIII, Factor IX and heparin.[45,46,47,48] However, unlike the differences between thromboplastins, the reasons for the different performance of APTT reagents are not well established. Opinions differ as to whether different types of activator are or are not[45,46] responsible for differences in heparin sensitivity while buffering of the phospholipid/activator mixture may also be important.[49] In an attempt to clarify the situation, studies have recently been carried out in our laboratory with the aim of establishing the most important determinants of reagent differences[50,51] and these are discussed in the following sections.

Activation method

The importance of standardizing the activation technique was emphasized by the studies of Lenahan and Phillips,[52] who showed that clotting times varied according to the concentration of activator and its reaction time with the plasma. These authors used Celite, but most laboratories now use kaolin as a particulate activator. This is stable but may differ between batches and it is recommended that a single large batch be purchased. In our own studies the use of Owren's buffer instead of saline as a diluent for both kaolin and phospholipid improved the sensitivity to heparin[51] and a buffered system is described in the standardized technique (Appendix II at end of chapter). The activation time is an important source of variability; times between one and 20 minutes have been reported. In platelet rich plasma 20 minutes is required for full activation and release of PF_3.[53] When phospholipid is used instead of platelets activation is completed more rapidly, and 10 minutes is optimal.[54] However, many manufacturers, and some coagulation textbooks, [55,56] recommend times of one to five minutes. In comparative studies of different reagents[47,48] activation times of two, three, four, five and six minutes were used, but it was not clear whether the reported differences in sensitivities were due to these activation differences, or different phospholipids, or both. In our studies, using the same phospholipid reagent, it was found that decreasing the activation time from 10 minutes reduced the sensitivity to Factor VIII.[50] The situation with heparin, however, was more complex[51] (Fig. 4.4). Because of the delaying effect of heparin on surface activation the prolongation of clotting times of the heparinized sample was much greater during the first few minutes than after 10 minutes, and maximum heparin sensitivity was obtained after two minutes' activation. However, such

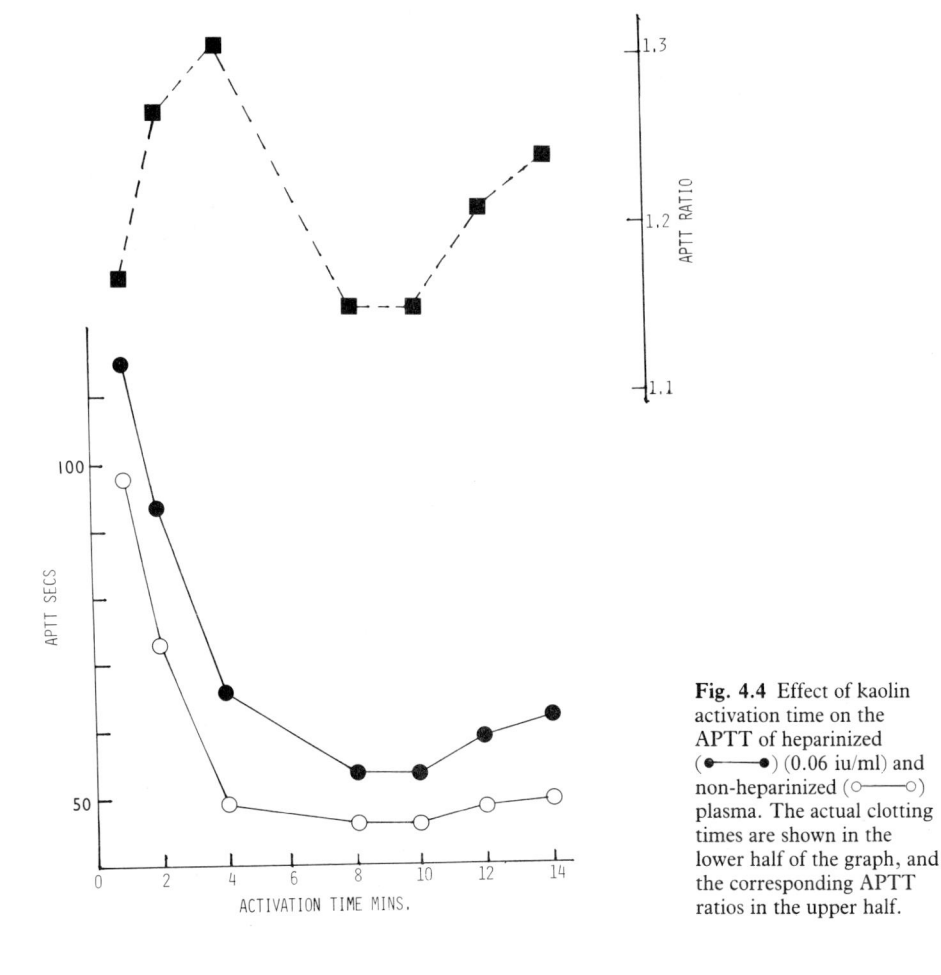

Fig. 4.4 Effect of kaolin activation time on the APTT of heparinized (●——●) (0.06 iu/ml) and non-heparinized (○——○) plasma. The actual clotting times are shown in the lower half of the graph, and the corresponding APTT ratios in the upper half.

suboptimal activation times cannot be recommended as the degree of activation at two minutes is likely to vary between individuals, and with different concentrations of heparin, will lead to poor linearity and precision. Overall, a 10-minute activation time with kaolin is preferable for standardization since it gives full activation of the non-heparinized plasma.

The advent of automatic coagulometers has caused some problems with the APTT because of the tendency of kaolin to settle out. A liquid activator of Factor XII, ellagic acid[57], has been incorporated into several commercial reagents. The ellagic acid is combined with the phospholipid in a stable emulsion giving a single reagent which simplifies the technique. However, in a number of comparative studies the ellagic acid reagents have been among the least sensitive to intrinsic factor deficiencies and heparin[58,59] though it was not clear whether the ellagic acid or phospholipid was responsible. In our studies the use of ellagic acid instead of kaolin as activator with the same phospholipid considerably reduced its sensitivity to heparin.[51] If ellagic acid is used the activation time can be shortened from 10 minutes; for one of the reagents (Cephotest) six minutes was found to be the optimum time.[60] A non-settling, particulate activator (micronized silica) suitable for automatic coagulometers is claimed to give improved sensitivity over ellagic acid.[49]

Phospholipid

The chemical and physical characteristics of phospholipid preparations required for their optimum procoagulant activity have been the subject of much investigation.[61,62] The presence of unsaturated fatty acids and a net negative charge on the molecule seem to be the basic requirements for activity. Although there are no species effects, differences in tissue source and extraction method give phospholipids of different composition and the procoagulant activity is also affected by the method used for emulsification.

Because most laboratories use commercial reagents the onus of standardization of extraction methods is on the manufacturers. However, a number of laboratories still prefer to make their own phospholipid reagents, using methods such as that described by Denson[55] and Giddings.[56] Because of their high content of unsaturated fatty acids phospholipids are very susceptible to oxidative degradation. This may arise during preparation and storage and precautions should be taken against oxidation. A modified method of preparation has been used in our laboratory with the aim of minimizing oxidative changes and producing a stable reagent (see Appendix IV).[63] The optimum dilution of such home-made reagents should be determined carefully using normal, factor-deficient and heparinized plasmas. If the optimum dilution changes over a period of time this indicates instability and a new batch should be prepared.

A study of the most commonly used reagents indicated that several were partially oxidized.[50] Oxidation of phospholipids produces compounds which themselves affect clotting times[64] and therefore alters their procoagulant characteristics. Controlled oxidation of a phospholipid reagent did not affect its ability to detect Factor VIII deficiency, but did alter its sensitivity to heparin.

A 70-fold range of total organic phosphorus concentration was found amongst commercial reagents[50] although not all the extractable phosphorus need represent procoagulant phospholipid. Our own studies showed that, whilst a wide range of phospholipid concentrations were equally effective in detecting Factor VIII deficiency, the sensitivity of the APTT to heparin was affected by relatively small changes in phospholipid concentration. The sensitivity increased with decreasing concentration.[50,51]

Approaches to standardization

The number of variables in the APTT is considerably more than in the prothrombin time, and progress towards national and international standardization has been limited. In the UK, a standard cephalin extract[54] has been incorporated in proficiency assessment surveys run by the NRLARC since 1974. The standardized reagent was found to be superior to most commercial reagents in detecting intrinsic factor deficiencies.[65,66] Similarly, the standardized reagent showed greater sensitivity to heparin, both in the proficiency trials and in an international study.[59] An important feature of the NRLARC reagent is that the technique is also standardized and this is reproduced in detail in Appendix II in the end of this chapter.

The NRLARC reagent is now available for routine use. There is no doubt that, as for the PT, adoption of a single reagent and standardized technique on a national scale is the simplest, most direct way of standardizing the APTT. However, such a system is impracticable in many countries. From a US survey reported in 1977[17,67] it was found that seven different reagents and 11 different clot detection methods were used, giving 77 possible combinations. However, only 20 of these were in common use, with 10 systems accounting for more than 70 per cent of laboratories. The educational effect of such surveys may account for the fact that over 50 per cent of the laboratories in the US survey used three of the most precise combinations.

The problems of standardization of the APTT should be kept in perspective. For the intrinsic clotting factor deficiencies quantitation is carried out by specific assays. It is necessary only for the APTT to be sensitive to the lowest reduction in clotting factor concentrations likely to cause bleeding problems. Because of the reported differences in sensitivity of various reagents a study of the efficiency of reagents in detection of mild hemophilia was carried out.[68] Most reagents were able to distinguish clinically significant mild hemophilia from normal and none of the reagents was obviously superior to the others. Standardization of the APTT presents particular problems for the control of heparin therapy because of the attempts to define a therapeutic range in terms of APTT ratios. A range of one-and-a-half to two-and-a-half times the normal APTT[69] is widely quoted; this corresponded to a two- to three-times prolonged whole blood clotting time.[70] However, the use of such figures with different reagents than that originally used is invalid.[71,72] Comparison of different APTT reagents with a reference reagent gives poor correlation so that the system adopted by WHO for the PT is unlikely to work. However, the concentration of heparin can be determined by other methods. Thus, if a therapeutic range of heparin concentrations could be agreed, it would be a simple matter for each manufacturer to determine the APTT ratios of his reagent equivalent to this range. It is clear from recent reviews[73,74] that such a concensus has not yet been reached. An additional problem is that many patients undergoing heparin therapy are hypercoagulable, with baseline APTTs below normal, and the relationship between APTT ratio and heparin concentration may be quite different from that in normal plasma.

STANDARDIZATION OF SPECIFIC ASSAYS

Although the assays for specific clotting factors are generally more complex than the screening tests, their standardization is more straightforward. They differ from the screening tests in two important ways. First, the assay methods are designed to be specific for the clotting factor being measured. Secondly, in most cases concentrations of clotting factors are measured not as absolute values but by comparison with a reference standard. This system of comparison of an unknown sample with a reference material has the great advantage that changes in the test system, will affect both standard and unknown alike. However, different results can be given by different methods of measuring the same factor, even when the same reference standards are used. Such differences indicate a lack of complete specificity of the assay methods.

GENERAL PRINCIPLES OF CLOTTING ASSAYS

Normal plasma as a standard

Most components of the coagulation system were assayed before these substances were available in a pure form and the first 'standard' was simply normal plasma. The unit of activity for most clotting factors was defined as the amount in 1 ml 'average fresh normal plasma'. This system of standardization has a number of advantages. The standard is easy to obtain, contains the substances being measured in a state close to that of native blood and requires no purification. However, 'normal plasma' is hard to define because of differences associated with sex, race, age and blood group,[75] as well as the influence of drugs such as oral contraceptives. This intrinsic variability can cause appreciable differences in the activity of even large multi-donor pools. A further problem is the instability of some clotting factors, notably Factors V and VIII, on storage of plasma.

Stable reference standards

Greater uniformity in the measurement of biological activity has been achieved through the establishment of long-term reference standards of proven stability. Reference standards, which are usually freeze-dried, can either be plasmas or purified preparations and are not restricted to products derived from blood (e.g. heparin). The value of these materials does not lie in any particular attribute, e.g. purity (indeed, in many cases they are quite impure), but in the distillation of many assay results into a single figure which is accepted as the activity of the standard.

To use the standard as a 'yardstick' for measuring biological activity it must

```
                    INTERNATIONAL STANDARD
                      ╱              ╲
                     ╱                ╲
                    ╱                  ╲
                   ▼                    ▼
         NATIONAL STANDARD  ────▶  LOCAL STANDARD
                    ╲                  ╱
                     ╲                ╱
                      ▼              ▼
                        TEST SAMPLES
```

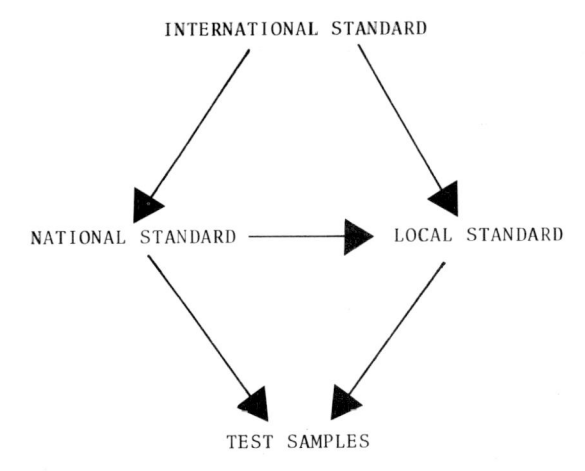

Fig. 4.5 The hierarchy of biological standardization. National standards are calibrated against the international standard. Local standards are calibrated against national standards or, where these do not exist, directly against the international standard. Test samples are assayed against either local or national standards.

be tested in an appropriate assay system in parallel with the preparation whose activity is to be measured. The result of the assay is an estimate of the relative activity, or *potency ratio* (R) of the preparation being tested, in terms of the standard. If the standard is defined to contain S units per ml, the unknown is then estimated to contain R × S units per ml. In practice, a single standard preparation cannot suffice as the standard in all assays, since it would rapidly be used up. Multiple standards are therefore necessary, and their relative potencies must be estimated if their activities are to be expressed in the same units. This is most efficiently done by designating one material as a primary (international) standard and reserving this exclusively for the calibration of secondary (national or laboratory) standards. In this way a hierarchy of quantitation may be established starting from the primary standard by which the unit is defined and ending with the various unknowns to be assayed (Fig. 4.5).

Table 4.5 gives a list of the international standards and reference preparations currently available in the area of hemostasis and thrombosis. Measurement of all these materials can now be made in international units by reference to the appropriate standard. For some frequently assayed factors national standards have also been developed; these are calibrated against the appropriate international standard. For instance, in the UK, national standards have been developed for assay of Factor VIII, both in patients' plasma samples and in therapeutic concentrates. Where no national standards are available it may be necessary for individual laboratories to calibrate their own 'house standards' directly against the international standard.

Use of controls

Although the inclusion of control samples would appear to be a means of internal quality control, in practice it is less useful than in the case of the screening tests. If two samples are included in an assay, one of known and the

Table 4.5 International standards and reference materials in hemostasis and thrombosis.

Substance	Current Std.	Date established	Code No.
Human Factor VIII (concentrate)	2nd IS	1976	73/552
Human Factor IX (concentrate)	1st IS	1976	73/32
Thromboplastin (human brain)	1st IRP	1976	67/40
Thromboplastin (rabbit brain)	1st IRP	1976	70/178
Thromboplastin (bovine brain)	1st IRP	1976	68/434
Thrombin (human)	1st IS	1975	70/157
Plasmin (human)	1st IS	1976	72/379
Streptokinase	1st IS	1964	62/7
Urokinase	1st IRP	1966	66/46
Ancrod	1st IRP	1976	74/581
Heparin (porcine mucosal)	3rd IS	1973	65/69
Human antithrombin III (plasma)	1st IRP	1978	72/1

IS — International Standard
IRP — International Reference Preparation. (An IRP designation indicates that a material is suitable to serve as a reference preparation, but may require further characterization and collaborative studies before being accepted as an International Standard.)

All the above preparations are available from:
National Institute for Biological Standards and Control, Holly Hill, Hampstead, London NW3 6RB, UK.

other of unknown potency, the correctness of the result on the known sample has very little bearing on the result for the unknown sample. For instance, if standard and control samples are freeze-dried the same error of reconstitution may be made for both. This may give the 'right' result for the control but an incorrect potency for the unknown fresh plasma sample. A further problem is that the potency of commercially available control samples is usually only determined against the manufacturer's own standard with a single assay method. Laboratories using different standards and assay methods may not always obtain the same results.

In general, there is no simple method of ensuring that the result of a bioassay is the 'right' result. All assays have an intrinsic error and the best way to minimize this error is by repetition — replication within the assay — or a repeat of the whole assay for important measurements. The use of control samples is best restricted to answering specific questions, such as whether two operators, or two different methods of clot detection, are giving the same results. Appropriate statistical methods of calculating the activity of a plasma sample are an equally important part of the assay procedure.[76,77]

STANDARDIZATION OF SPECIFIC CLOTTING FACTORS

FACTOR VIII

Factor VIII is one of the most frequently assayed of the clotting factors; at least 25 000 assays are carried out annually in the UK,[78] mainly in connection with the control of hemophilia therapy. In the early days of treatment with plasma and cryoprecipitate local standardization with a normal pool was probably adequate. The problem of normal plasma as a standard is accentuated for Factor VIII because of its very wide normal range (50 to 200 per cent of average normal) and instability in plasma. With the advent of freeze-dried concentrates of Factor VIII it became clear that local standardization was inadequate. Wide divergences were shown to exist in the concept of 'average normal plasma' in different laboratories.[79] Two-stage assay methods were also generally more precise than the one-stage.[79] Freeze-dried Factor VIII concentrate was found to be stable and, because of its similarity to freeze-dried concentrates being used for therapy, a concentrate was chosen as the 1st international standard (IS) for Factor VIII.[80] The standard was assayed by comparison with fresh normal plasma in the 20 participating laboratories, a total of 167 donors, and assigned a value of 2.6 'normal plasma units' per ampoule; this became 2.6 International Units.

Assays of concentrates

All major manufacturers of Factor VIII concentrates now assay their products in international units, i.e. directly or indirectly against the IS. The IS for Factor VIII is intended as the primary reference preparation, and intermediate standards, national or local, must be used for assays of batches of concentrate (Fig. 4.5). Because calibration of one standard against another is subject to error it is best if the path between the IS and the samples for assay be made as short as possible. In the UK this has been achieved by the adoption of a common standard, the British Working Standard for Factor VIII Concentrate, by the production laboratories and by the National Institute for Biological Standards and Control (NIBSC). This concentrate standard is carefully calibrated against the IS by all laboratories using it. It is then used directly as a working standard in the assay of production batches.

In the US, each manufacturer has his own 'house standard' and, until recently, these have been calibrated against the US standard, issued by the FDA Bureau of Biologics (BoB) which is in turn calibrated against the IS. This 'double calibration' has led to discrepancies, with potencies of most manufacturers' products being 15 to 25 per cent higher against the BoB standard than when assayed directly against the IS. The causes of these discrepancies have been difficult to establish, but are probably related to the fact that the BoB standard is a plasma whereas the IS and the therapeutic materials are concentrates. It has now been agreed that the US manufacturers of concentrates will calibrate their working standards directly against the IS, instead of indirectly via the BoB standard.

It is preferable for manufacturers of concentrates to use samples of their own product as a working standard; in both the calibration process and the assay of production batches, 'like' is then being assayed against 'like'. Calibration of such working standards should be carried out carefully, with a minimum of six assays against the IS to obtain adequate precision. Although Factor VIII appears to be very stable in concentrates, the potency of working standards should be checked annually against the IS if they are going to be used for much longer than one year.

The first IS for Factor VIII was replaced in 1977 by the second IS, a similar intermediate purity concentrate. The new IS was compared with the first and also with samples of fresh normal plasma.[81] The relationship between the IU and average normal plasma was found to have remained reasonably constant and the new standard was assigned a potency of 1.1 IU per ampoule.[82] One of the main findings of this study was that when samples of a common freeze-dried plasma were assayed against the IS (concentrate) the two-stage assays gave significantly lower potencies than the one-stage assays. This finding, which was later shown to be a general phenomenon,[83] has far-reaching implications for the standardization of Factor VIII, particularly in the calibration of plasma standards and in the assessment of recovery.

Plasma standards

The standardization of Factor VIII assays in plasma has been more problematical than standardization of concentrates. Standardization of local pools can only be achieved by comparison with an external reference standard and, in principle, each local standard could be assayed against the IS. However, because of the large number of laboratories involved this is wasteful of resources and some sort of regional or national scheme is preferable. The UK system[84] is based on national plasma standards issued from NIBSC after calibration against the IS by several laboratories. A major problem with this system has been the occurrence of up to twofold discrepancies between different laboratories' potency estimates.[11] These discrepancies are of two kinds. First, there is a general discrepancy between one-stage and two-stage assays, the one-stage methods giving higher potencies for the plasma standards by an average of 20 per cent.[83] In addition, within each method there are differences between laboratories due to variations in reagents and techniques. Both these types of discrepancy arise from the dissimilar nature of the materials (plasma and concentrate) and are not seen when one plasma standard is compared against another. It is clear that the calibration of plasma standards against the IS (concentrate) is unsatisfactory in the long term and it has been decided to establish an international reference plasma for Factor VIII, to co-exist alongside the concentrate standard. As a result of improvements in methods of collection and freeze-drying, such a standard should have a lifetime of at least five years.[11] The 1st International Reference Preparation for Factor VIII Plasma will shortly be established[85] and has been calibrated by comparison with a large number of normal plasma samples.[86] Values for the other Factor VIII related activities have been determined in the standard, in addition to its Factor VIII clotting activity. The British plasma standard for Factor VIII will in future will be calibrated against the international plasma standard instead of the international concentrate standard. This should minimize the discrepancies between laboratories and avoid the need to assign an unsatisfactory compromise figure for the potency. Limitations of supply will mean that some larger laboratories have to use their own local standard, calibrated by reference to the British Standard. Although this is less preferable, it still ensures reasonable homogeneity of measurement of Factor VIII among all laboratories using the British Standard.

Some UK laboratories prefer to use commercial plasma standards. These are calibrated against either a local pool or the international standard (concentrate), but usually by the manufacturer's methods alone. There is no co-ordination between different manufacturers. This is a particular problem in the USA where several brands of commercial plasma standard are widely used and no national working standard is available. It is hoped that the establishment of the international plasma standard for Factor VIII will lead to greater uniformity through manufacturers being persuaded to use it for calibration of their plasma standards.

Standardization of reagents and techniques

Factor VIII in a test sample is always measured in comparison with a standard so that the influence of reagents and technical factors is less crucial than in the case of the screening tests. Nonetheless, the importance of reagents as a cause of interlaboratory discrepancy cannot be ignored. It has been found that the differences between laboratories using variations of the same method (one-stage or two-stage) were eliminated when all used the same reagents, although a difference between one-stage and two-stage methods remained.[87] This was particularly so when a combined freeze-dried reagent (prepared by mixing large batches of activated serum, phospholipid and Factor V, and freeze-drying the mixture) was used for the two-stage assays. Such combined reagents have been used in our laboratory for the past four years[88] and have proved helpful in internal quality control, avoiding day-to-day differences in serum activation and the need for frequent changes of batches (see Appendix V). It appears that the reagents are stable for at least a year. In the one-stage assays standardization of either the phospholipid or hemophilic plasma separately did not substantially improve interlaboratory agreement[11] and other influences, such as the activation method, may also be important. For internal quality control Factor VIII-deficient substrate plasma should be collected from several hemophiliacs, all with less than one per cent detectable Factor VIII activity.

The causes of the one-stage/two-stage discrepancy have not been easy to identify. A collaborative study was set up to investigate possible courses. Omission of the aluminium hydroxide ($Al(OH)_3$) adsorption step from the two-stage method reduced the discrepancy to less than 10 per cent.[89] However, the two-stage assay technique without adsorption is not entirely satisfactory for clinical samples, and further studies are in progress on other modifications of the adsorption technique. In vivo studies showed that the one-stage assays have recoveries of approximately 100 per cent, whereas the two-stage method gave about 80 per cent recovery.[90] At present, it is not possible to say which method, if either, is 'correct'.

Proficiency assessment

Samples for Factor VIII assay have only recently been included in proficiency assessment trials. The first survey in the USA of 530 laboratories showed considerable variability of results, with coefficients of variation ranging from 55.5 to 76.5 per cent on the mild hemophilic plasma sample (around 10 per cent Factor VIII) and somewhat less for the normal plasma.[91] About two-thirds of the laboratories used a variety of commercial standards; the remainder used local plasma pools. It was concluded that the different standards used were the main source of variability. In the UK, samples for Factor VIII assay have recently been included in the NRLARC proficiency assessment scheme and it will be interesting to see whether the availability of a common standard has influenced the overall precision as compared with the US results.

FACTOR IX AND OTHER CLOTTING FACTORS

Many of the problems of standardization of Factor VIII apply also to Factor IX. A stable reference standard is needed for assay of the therapeutic concentrates used for treatment of Factor IX deficiency, and in an international collaborative study freeze-dried concentrate and plasma samples were compared with samples of fresh normal plasma.[92] Factor IX is more stable than Factor VIII, and the plasma sample in this study was only slightly less stable than the concentrate. The concentrate was established as the 1st international standard for Factor IX with 5.6 IU per ampoule.[93] As with Factor VIII, 'like against like' gives greatest precision, and concentrate working standards are preferable for assay of therapeutic materials. In the UK a British working standard for Factor IX concentrate is calibrated against the IS and used by the production laboratories and by NIBSC. UK plasma standards have also been calibrated against the IS for Factor IX; for the last few batches the practice has been to use the same plasma standard for both Factor VIII and Factor IX. However, the pre-dilution method used for the concentrate is an important source of variability; using Factor IX-deficient plasma instead of buffer as a pre-diluent for the IS can alter the potency of the plasma by as much as 50 per cent.[94] With Factor IX-deficient plasma as a pre-diluent, the potencies of the plasma standards are lower (around 0.6 IU/ampoule) than would be obtained by assay against normal pooled plasmas. However, this method has been adopted as it gives a value which is more consistent with the post-infusion samples obtained after injection of concentrate into Factor IX-deficient patients.

As yet no international standards have been established for clotting factors other than VIII or IX, and the laboratory must rely on commercial standards or local pools. The other clotting factors have narrower normal ranges than Factor VIII and, with the exception of Factor V, are more stable. A pool of normal plasma will generally provide adequate standardization. This should be derived from at least 20 subjects who are not taking drugs known to affect clotting factors, e.g. anticoagulants, oral contraceptives, and whose age range should not be narrowly confined. Plasma should be centrifuged immediately after collection, snap-frozen and stored at as low a temperature as possible, preferably −70°C or below.

FIBRINOGEN

A variety of different methods have evolved for the measurement of fibrinogen based on its ability to form a clot. Measurement of the tyrosine content of a carefully collected and washed clot[95] is widely regarded as a reference method. The thrombin clotting time is best used only as a comparative assay against a fibrinogen standard. Plasmas of known fibrinogen content are available commercially.

Samples for fibrinogen assay have been included in the NRLARC proficiency assessment scheme since 1976. The most popular methods are the fibrinogen titre and the Clauss thrombin time method. All techniques performed reasonably well with fibrinogen levels in the normal range but for low fibrinogen levels the thrombin time method tended to differ from the others. The turbidity technique, fibrinogen titre and heat precipitation methods were also relatively unreliable.

Similar variability in type of method and results was reported in the US from the early proficiency assessment studies of the College of American Pathologists, with coefficients of variation for all methods ranging from 21 to 90 per cent. However, since 1971 the thrombin time method introduced by Dade has become very popular, and is now preferred by more than 80 per cent of laboratories in the US. This method, based on comparison against a standard, has given much improved accuracy and precision with overall coefficients of variation in the region of 5 to 10 per cent in the 1978 survey.[96]

THROMBIN

Although assays of thrombin are rarely carried out for clinical purposes, thrombin is widely used as a reagent, and it is important that its measurement be standardized. An international standard for human thrombin is available[97] and all manufacturers of diagnostic reagents are encouraged to calibrate their thrombin against it, using a comparative bioassay method. No consistent differences were reported in precision and potency estimates when plasma or fibrinogen, from either bovine or human sources, were used as substrate.[97]

ANTITHROMBIN III

The recognition that a congenital or acquired deficiency of antithrombin III (At III), can be a major predisposing factor in the development of thrombosis has led to increased interest in the measurement of this inhibitor.[98] This interest has also been stimulated by the introduction of synthetic peptide substrates for measurement of thrombin and other enzymes, which has simplified the technique and improved the precision of At III assays. Results are sometimes expressed as 'inhibitor units' instead of the more usual percentage activity in comparison with a normal plasma standard. These 'inhibitor units' are defined in terms of the amount of thrombin inhibited under certain specified reaction conditions. The difficulty of reproducing the conditions exactly and the basic biological variability of the system make this an unreliable method of standardization. If this method is used it is essential to compare the inhibitor units given by the test sample with a standard curve prepared with the same reagents. Another common practice is to assay test sample at a single dilution only, usually in duplicate. Such single point estimates have a high intrinsic error, and economic savings should be weighed against the clinical consequences that may result from a false estimate. Ideally, three dilutions of test samples should be measured but if only two measurements are possible it is better that these be of two independent dilutions in different parts of the standard curve rather than duplicates from the same single dilution. Although the precision will probably be less than with duplicates the mean value will be a truer assessment of the At III level.

A study has recently carried out with the aim of establishing a stable reference standard.[99] Samples of highly purified At III and freeze-dried plasma were compared with local pooled plasma in 11 laboratories. Considerable discrepancies were found between the different assay methods when the purified At III samples were assayed against the common freeze-dried plasma. In contrast, comparison of the freeze-dried plasma with local pools gave remarkably good agreement between different methods. The plasma was also more stable than the purified materials and the freeze-dried plasma was chosen as the 1st international reference preparation for At III. It is intended for calibration of both local and commercial standards though, as with Factor VIII, a regional or national standardization scheme is preferable. In the UK, batches of British plasma standard for Factor VIII have also been calibrated for At III, so that laboratories can use it as a working standard for both substances.

HEPARIN

Although heparin is not a clotting factor its concentration can only be assessed by its interaction with various components of the plasma coagulation system, notably At III. The method of measurement of heparin by its effect on the APTT has already been discussed. An alternative assay for heparin which is claimed to be more specific is the anti-Xa assay.[100,101] In this method, the clotting times obtained are compared with a standard curve prepared by in vitro addition of heparin dilutions to plasma, thus enabling an estimate of heparin concentration to be made. In principle, comparison against a standard curve can be made for any heparin test, including the APTT, but the anti-Xa method is less likely to be affected by varying concentrations of clotting factors in the plasma.

The essential point to appreciate in measuring heparin concentration, by whatever method, is the very wide variability in the response of different indi-

Table 4.6 Heparin sensitivity by APTT in different subjects.

Subject	CT (s) at 0.2 iu/ml	Heparin IU/ml at APTT ratio of 2
1	136	0.11
2	110	0.15
3	96	0.17
4	114	0.12
5	73	0.20
6	82	0.13

Table 4.7 Clotting times and heparin concentrations by APTT after i.v. injection of 1000 IU heparin into six subjects.

Subject	APTT (Secs.)	Heparin concentration IU/ml Pooled plasma	Pre-injection plasma
1	90	0.20	0.115
2	66	0.11	0.093
3	72	0.14	0.12
4	58.3	0.08	0.06
5	102	0.24	0.14
6	99.5	0.23	0.15

Heparin concentrations were estimated by comparing APTTs to standard curves prepared in either pooled normal plasma or each subject's pre-injection plasma.

viduals to in vitro addition of the same heparin concentration. Table 4.6 shows the variability in APTT clotting times obtained on addition of 0.2 IU/ml heparin to the plasma of six individuals in our laboratory. Thus an APTT ratio of two corresponds to a twofold range of heparin concentrations. Similar differences between individuals are seen in the anti-Xa assay. From study of different individuals, this degree of variation in sensitivity to heparin is not atypical, and may be even greater in patients' plasmas. It is common practice to assess the heparin concentration in test plasmas by reference to a standard curve prepared in pooled normal plasma. It can be seen from Table 4.6 that this could result in substantial error in measurement of heparin concentration. This is shown in Table 4.7, where values obtained from a standard curve in pooled plasma are compared with values obtained from standard curves prepared in each subject's pre-injection plasma. Whilst the practical difficulties of obtaining pre-injection plasma from patients are appreciated, comparison with standard curves in pre-injection plasma is nonetheless the only satisfactory way of obtaining a reliable estimate of heparin concentration.

Even when measured in this way, heparin concentrations given by the various assay methods do not always agree. As can be seen from Table 4.8, there is a tendency for the anti-Xa method to give higher values than the APTT. The reasons for this are complex, but one important finding is that after injection of heparin anti-Xa values are increased by a component which is not neutralisable

Table 4.8 Comparison of heparin concentrations by APTT and anti-Xa assays after i.v. injection of 1000 IU heparin into six subjects.

Subject	Heparin IU/ml Anti-Xa	APTT
1	0.20	0.115
2	0.22	0.093
3	0.17	0.12
4	0.16	0.06
5	0.23	0.14
6	0.19	0.15
Mean	0.19	0.11

All heparin concentrations were determined from standard curves made with each subject's pre-injection plasma.

by protamine sulphate or platelet factor 4,[102] and therefore is not heparin. The nature of this 'extra' anti-Xa activity is poorly understood, but it appears to be much less when anti-Xa is measured by a chromogenic substrate. This latter method therefore probably gives the truest estimate of heparin concentration. The key question which has not been answered is whether the antithrombotic effect of heparin is related to its concentration in the blood or to its overall effect on clotting as measured by the APTT. The main point to bear in mind is that, without adequate standardization both types of measurement can be subject to gross error.

APPENDIX I: PROTHROMBIN TIME TEST (reproduced with kind permission from Thomson[2])

Collection of blood
Collect venous blood using a polystyrene syringe fitted with a 20 or 21 G needle into a suitable, capped plastic vessel containing a freshly prepared solution of 3.13 per cent trisodium citrate, $Na_3C_6H_5O_7 2H_2O$. (One volume of anticoagulant to nine volumes of blood.) Mix by gentle inversion several times.

It is advisable to store containers, for blood collection, upright and preferably in a rack at 4°C. A system should be instituted to ensure that the citrate anticoagulant is always used fresh and the containers are discarded if not used within a certain time to avoid the chance of loss of anticoagulant due to evaporation.

Separation of plasma
Centrifuge blood as soon as possible after collection to obtain platelet-poor plasma (1500 to 2000 g for 15 min). Using a siliconed pasteur pipette, transfer plasma to a second non-wettable container. Store at 4°C in crushed ice. Plasma samples should be tested as soon as possible and not more than two hours after collection.

Performance of test

Reagents
Calcium chloride 0.025 M. Prepare from a M/1 solution.

Glassware
Use chemically clean, unscratched glass tubes. Finely calibrated 0.1 ml pipettes (E-MIL type) should be used.

Method
Into a waterbath at 37°C place to warm:
a. Sufficient glass tubes for testing samples.
b. An aliquot of calcium chloride (0.025 M).
Into a glass tube add:

1. 0.1 ml thromboplastin ⎫ Warm together for one
2. 0.1 ml plasma ⎭ to two min.
3. 0.1 ml calcium chloride solution

Start stop-watch. Tilt evenly and gently until clot is formed. The speed and angle of tilting of the test tube should be standardized, to minimize the cooling caused by withdrawal from 37°C waterbath. Tilting × 3 every 5 s, through an angle of 90°, is recommended. Excessive cooling may result in a prolongation of the prothrombin time. Tests should be performed in duplicate. If the discrepancy between duplicate tests is more than five per cent of the mean clotting time, both should be repeated, e.g. if the mean clotting time is 30 seconds, duplicates should range between 28.5 and 31.5 seconds.

When performing a calibration procedure to test the sensitivity of a test thromboplastin compared with a reference thromboplastin, the order of testing each individual plasma, in duplicate, should be as follows:

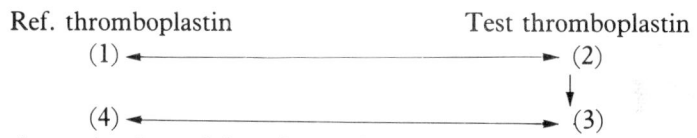

```
        Ref. thromboplastin           Test thromboplastin
              (1) ←————————————————————→ (2)
                                           ↓
              (4) ←————————————————————— (3)
```

i.e. each plasma is pipetted into four tubes and tested with the two thromboplastin extracts, in duplicate. Do not pipette more than one plasma at a time into test tube warming in waterbath.

APPENDIX II: ACTIVATED PARTIAL THROMBOPLASTIN TIME (APTT) USING STANDARDIZED CEPHALIN REAGENT (reproduced with kind permission from Thomson[2])

Reagents

1. Standardized cephalin reagent*. Store vials of lyophilized extract at −20°C. Reconstitute with 1.0 ml distilled water and gently agitate for one or two minutes, by hand, to suspend. This stock suspension may be stored for several months at −20°C. It may be thawed and refrozen on numerous occasions to obtain an aliquot for a working suspension, provided that the thawing is performed rapidly and its temperature is not allowed to rise above 4°C. It should be returned rapidly to a temperature of −20°C immediately after sampling. Prepare a working suspension immediately before use, by diluting an aliquot of the stock suspension 1:50 in Owren's buffer, i.e. 0.1 ml cephalin, 4.9 ml Owren's buffer, in a plastic test-tube or container. Maintain in crushed ice. Discard after one hour.

2. Owren's buffer: dissolve 11.75 g of sodium diethylbarbiturate and 14.67 g of NaCl in a mixture of 1570 ml distilled water and 430 ml of 0.1 N HCl (pH 7.35).

3. Calcium chloride (0.025 M).
4. Light kaolin, suspended in Owren's buffer (0.5 g/100 ml).
5. Dilution fluid, i.e. 200 ml Owren's buffer
                   200 ml sodium citrate (0.025 M)
                   600 ml 0.9 per cent w/v NaCl

* Obtainable, on request, from National (UK) Reference Laboratory for Anticoagulant Reagents and Control, Withington Hospital, Manchester M20 8LR, UK.

Method
Collect blood using a polystyrene syringe fitted with a 20 or 21 G needle into 3.13 per cent tri-sodium citrate ($Na_3C_6H_5O_7 2H_2O$) in a plastic container (nine volumes blood, one volume anti-coagulant). Centrifuge immediately for 15 min at 2000 g. If plasma is hemolyzed, collect fresh sample if possible. Decant plasma into plastic container, standing in crushed ice. Test plasmas as soon as possible and not later than one hour after collection.

Test
Place glass tubes for performance of test and tubes containing calcium chloride, kaolin suspension and dilution fluid to warm in waterbath at 37°C.
  Into warm glass clotting tube add:
0.2 ml dilution fluid
0.2 ml plasma
0.2 ml cephalin suspension
0.1 ml kaolin suspension
  Start stop-watch. Tilt tube × 3 to mix and subsequently tilt once at approximately one minute intervals, to resuspend kaolin. At exactly ten minutes, add 0.2 ml calcium chloride and tilt × 3 to mix. Leave undisturbed until stop-watch reads 30 seconds from time of recalcification then tilt tube gently until sold clot forms. Record clotting time from addition of calcium.
  Perform duplicate test on each plasma.
  Simultaneous tests can be performed by using several stop watches and phasing the start of tests by appropriate intervals.
  Normal range: 38 to 45 sec.

APPENDIX III: QUANTITATIVE COMPARISON OF THROMBOPLASTINS (method of Kirkwood[40])

Method
In this alternative method to the Biggs and Denson procedure results for the samples from individual patients and normal subjects are plotted as actual *prothrombin times* on a log scale. The vertical axis is used for the reference thromboplastin and the horizontal axis for the test reagent. A linear relationship of the form

is obtained, where
$Y = A + BX$
$Y = \log PT$ (ref thromboplastin)
$X = \log PT$ (test thromboplastin)
A = a constant
B = slope of line

A 'best fit' line can be drawn through the points by eye, or by a more statistically rigorous method such as orthogonal regression.[40] It should be noted that simple linear regression is not appropriate, as both X and Y are variables subject to error.

Calculation of PT ratios

Once the slope of the line B has been determined by the above method, the PT ratios (PTR) of test and reference thromboplastins are related as follows:

$$\log \text{PTR (ref)} = B \times \log \text{PTR (test)}$$

The slope of the line B is designated the calibration constant, though it must be stressed that its numerical value will be different from that determined by the Biggs and Denson procedure.

APPENDIX IV: PREPARATION OF STABLE PHOSPHOLIPID REAGENTS

Principles

One of the main causes of instability of phospholipid reagents is oxidative degradation of the unsaturated fatty acids. In this method degradation is minimized by the following procedures:
1. Acetone-dried powder is prepared from fresh brain. Stored powder should not be used.
2. All solvents (including acetone) should contain an antioxidant. A suitable antioxidant is butylated hydroxyanisole (BHA) at a concentration of 0.1 mM.
3. The extractions should be carried out within a day, and the reagent emulsion prepared as soon as possible after the phospholipid powder is dry.

Preparation of acetone-dried brain

Remove meninges and blood clots from brain, wash in ice-cold 0.15 NaCl, cut into small pieces and weigh. Homogenize in a Waring blender with 1 volume (1 vol = 1 ml/g) cold acetone, transfer to Buchner funnel and filter. Extract residue 3 times with 1 volume cold acetone. Transfer moist residue to flask and dry, first under vacuum, then by blowing with nitrogen. Process powder immediately by one of the following two methods.

Extraction according to Bell and Alton: Add 1 volume chloroform to acetone-dried powder and mix vigorously for 10 minutes. Remove undissolved material by filtration, and evaporate to dryness. Dry the phospholipid powder in vacuo and store in a vacuum desiccator at −20°C.

Extraction by modified Folch procedure: Add 1 volume petroleum ether (40–60) to acetone-dried powder, and mix vigorously for 10 minutes. Evaporate the filtrate to leave a moist powder, and dissolve this in 0.2 volumes diethyl ether. If necessary, remove undissolved material by filtration, then precipitate the phospholipid by the addition of 1 volume cold acetone. Filter, wash the precipitate with cold acetone, dry in vacuo and store in a vacuum desiccator at −20°C.

Preparation and standardization of reagents

Prepare an emulsion (using a Vortex or sonicator) in distilled water containing antioxidant (BHA is dissolved in a small volume of ethanol and dispersed in 1 litre of water to 0.1 mM concentration). 5–10 mg/ml is a suitable concentration.

This stock emulsion can be distributed into aliquots and stored, preferably freeze-dried under nitrogen at −20°C, alternatively frozen at −40°C or below. For testing activity, a range of dilutions from 1/10 to 1/1000 is tested in the APTT. The highest dilution giving the shortest clotting time is chosen. The sensitivity to heparin and Factor VIII should be checked, using plasmas containing 0.05 IU/ml heparin and 20–30 IU/dl Factor VIII. For comparison of sensitivity, reference reagents are available from NRLARC and NIBSC.

The Bell and Alton extract is suitable for APTT and one-stage assays, but the Folch extract is preferable for two-stage Factor VIII assays, and can also be used for the APTT and one-stage assays. For standardization of two-stage Factor VIII assays, see Appendix V.

APPENDIX V: PREPARATION OF STANDARDIZED COMBINED REAGENT FOR TWO-STAGE FACTOR VIII ASSAY

In this method, large batches of the three individual reagents (serum, Factor V and phospholipid) are prepared and characterized. The reagents are then combined in bulk, and aliquots of the mixture freeze-dried in ampoules or vials. Each vial then contains the same amount of combined reagent, and if large enough batches are used, the reagents are 'standardized' for periods of several months.

Reagents

Serum: Blood from several donors is collected in dry glass tubes, allowed to clot for 4 to 6 hours at 37°C, and the serum separated after overnight incubation at 4°C. After removal of chylomicra by centrifugation (2 h at 27000 g or more), 1 or 2 ml aliquots are stored frozen or freeze-dried in glass vials.

Factor V: Obtained commercially, from Diagnostic Reagents Ltd, Thame, Oxon.

Phospholipid: Prepared by modified Folch procedure (see Appendix IV)

Combination of reagents

The normal procedure is to investigate 'plateau' formation of Factor Xa with varying concentrations of each of the three reagents. However, on mixing and freeze-drying, a certain proportion of activity is lost, particulary from the activated serum and Factor V, and optimum concentrations are difficult to determine. A mixture which has given consistently reliable results in our laboratory is as follows (quantities can be scaled down accordingly):

Serum	—	80 × 1 ml vials
Factor V	—	80 vials
Phospholipid	—	10 × 1 ml vials (10 mg/ml)

Activate the serum by incubating at 1/10 dilution in imidazole buffer (pH 7.4), overnight at 4°C. (N.B. for optimum activation use individual vials rather than pooling serum in a beaker). On the following morning, reconstitute each vial of factor V and phospholipid in 1 ml water, and mix all three reagents in a beaker for approximately 15 minutes. Distribute the mixed reagent into approximately 650 vials and freeze-dry.

Use of the Combined Reagent

When prepared as above, each vial should be reconstituted in 5 ml water and is ready for immediate use in the assay. The reconstitution volume can be varied if the clotting times are unacceptably long or short. Blank clotting times should be greater than 40 seconds. The reagent can be used, in either the classical 'subsampling' method, or the 'nonsubsampling' method described by Denson[55]; in the latter case, a further 1/2 dilution of the reagent should be made. With both methods, normal blood bank plasma can be used as substrate in the second stage. When prepared as above, the combined reagent should be stable for at least 6 months; blank times and the slope of the standard curve can be used as indexes of the reagent's activity.

REFERENCES

1. Quick A J 1935 The prothrombin in haemophilia and in obstructive jaundice. Journal of Biological Chemistry 109: lxxiii–lxxiv
2. Thomson J M 1980 Laboratory control of anticoagulant therapy. In: Thomson J M (ed) Blood coagulation and haemostasis: a practical guide. Churchill Livingstone, Edinburgh, ch 9, p 279–330
3. Mannucci P M Mariani G, Tentori L 1980 Standardisation and Quality Control of Coagulation Tests Scandinavian Journal of Haematology: (Suppl 37) 25, 1–161
4. Triplett D A (ed) 1981 Standardisation of Coagulation Assays (to be published)
5. Poller L 1980 Quality control in blood coagulation. In: Thomson J M (ed) Blood coagulation and Haemostasis: a practical guide. Churchill Livingstone, Edinburgh, ch 10, p 331–359
6. Ingram G I C, Hills M 1976 The prothrombin time test: effect of varying citrate concentration. Thrombosis and Haemostasis 36: 230–236
7. Mibashan R (unpublished data)
8. Ingram G I C, Hills M 1976 ICTH reference method for the one stage prothrombin time test on human blood. Thrombosis and the Haemostasis 36: 237–238
9. Zucker S, Cathey M H, West B 1970 Preparation of quality control specimens for coagulation. American Journal of Clinical Pathology 53: 924–927
10. Godfrey R. Rhymes I L, Bidwell E, Barrowcliffe T W 1975 The buffering of anticoagulants for blood collection. Thrombosis et Diathesis Haemorrhagica 34: 879–882
11. Barrowcliffe T W, Kirkwood T B L 1980 Standardization of Factor VIII. I: Calibration of British Standards for Factor VIII clotting activity. British Journal of Haemotology 46: 471–481
12. Jackson C M, Suttie J W 1977 Recent developments in understanding the mechanism of vitamin K and vitamin K-antagonist drug action and the consequences of vitamin K action in blood coagulation. Progress in Haematology 10: 333–359
13. Hemker H C, Veltkamp J J, Loeliger E A 1968 Kinetic aspects of the interaction of blood clotting enzymes. III: Demonstration of an inhibitor of prothrombin conversion in vitamin K deficiency. Thrombosis et Diathesis Haemorrhagica 19: 346–363
14. Hemker H C, Müller A D, Loeliger E A 1970 Two types of prothrombin in vitamin K deficiency. Thrombosis et Diathesis Haemorrhagica 23: 633–637
15. Jackson C M 1977 Recommended nomenclature for blood clotting zymogens and zymogen activation products of the International Committee on Thrombosis and Haemostasis. Thrombosis and Haemostasis 38: 567–577
16. Allen E V 1947 The clinical use of anticoagulants. Journal of the American Medical Association 134: 323–329

17. Koepke J 1977 Evaluation of materials and methods for coagulation testing. In: Henry J B, Giegel J L (eds) Quality control in laboratory medicine. Masson, New York, p 157–166
18. Poller L, Thomson J M, Yee K F 1978 Automated versus manual techniques for the prothrombin time test: results of proficiency assessment studies. British Journal of Haematology 38: 391–399
19. Loeliger E A 1979 The optimal therapeutic range in oral anticoagulation. History and proposal. Thrombosis and Haemostasis 42: 1141–1152
20. Biggs R 1965 Report on the standardisation of the one-stage prothrombin time for the control of anticoagulant therapy. In: Hunter R B, Wright I S, Koller F, Streuli F (eds) Genetics and the interaction of blood clotting factors. Thrombosis et Diathesis Haemorrhagica 17: Suppl, p 303–307
21. Goguel A 1976 Contrôle de qualité du temps de Quick. Renseignements formis par les confrontations interlaboratoires 'Etalonorme' 1973 à 1975. Feullets de Biologie 17: 31–42
22. Lam-Po-Tang P R L C, Poller L 1975 Oral anticoagulant therapy and its control: an international survey. Thrombosis et Diathesis Haemorrhagica 34: 419–425
23. Biggs R, Denson K W E 1967 Standardization of the one-stage prothrombin time for the control of anticoagulant therapy. British Medical Journal 1: 84–88
24. Poller L, Ingram G I C 1975 Standardisation and quality control of anticoagulant control. In: Lewis S M, Carter J F (eds) Quality control in haematology. Academic Press, London, ch 13, p 153–169
25. Leck I, Gowland E, Poller L 1974 The variability of measurements of prothrombin time ratio in the National Quality Control Trials — a follow-up study. British Journal of Haematology 28: 601–612
26. Poller L, Thomson J M, Yee K F 1979 Quality control trials of the prothrombin time: an assessment of the performance in serial studies. Journal of Clinical Pathology 32: 251–253
27. Loeliger E A, Halem-Visser L P van 1975 A simplified thromboplastin calibration procedure for standardization of anticoagulant control. Thrombosis et Diathesis Haemorrhagica 33: 172–190
28. Dijk-Wierda C A van, Hermans J, Loeliger E A, Roos J 1977 Interlaboratory oral anticoagulant quality assessment by the Netherlands Federation of Thrombosis Services. Thrombosis and Haemostasis 37: 509
29. Bain B, Forster T, Sleigh B 1978 Control of oral anticoagulants by the prothrombin time: a plea for uniformity. Medical Journal of Australia 2: 459–461
30. Miale J B, la Fond D J 1969 Prothrombin time standardisation. American Journal of Clinical Pathology 52: 154–160
31. Miale J B, Kent J W 1972 Standardization of the therapeutic range for oral anticoagulants based on standard reference plasmas. American Journal of Clinical Pathology 57: 80–88
32. Brozović M, Gurd L J, Robertson I, Bangham D R 1971 Stability of prothrombin and factor VII in freeze-dried plasma. Journal of Clinical Pathology 24: 690–693
33. Brozović M, Gurd L J, Robertson I, Bangham D R 1971 Factor X in freeze-dried factor VIII reference plasma. British Journal of Haematology 21: 201–208
34. Loeliger E A, Halem-Visser L P van 1979 Biological properties of the thromboplastins and plasmas included in the ICTH/ICSH collaborative study on prothrombin time standardization. Thrombosis and Haemostasis 42: 1115–1117
35. Koepke J A, Gilmer P R Jr, Triplett D A, O'Sullivan M B 1977 The prediction of prothrombin time performance using secondary standards. American Journal of Clinical Pathology 68: 191–194
36. Bangham D R, Biggs R, Brozović M, Denson K W E 1970 Draft report of a collaborative study of two thromboplastins (including the use of common abnormal plasmas). Thrombosis et diathesis Haemorrhagica, Suppl 40: 341–351
37. Denson K W E 1971 International and national standardization of control of anticoagulant therapy in patients receiving coumarin and indanedione drugs using calibrated thromboplastin preparations. Journal of Clinical Pathology 24: 460–463
38. Bangham D R, Biggs R, Brozović M, Denson K W E 1973 Calibration of five different thromboplastins, using fresh and freeze-dried plasma. Thrombosis et Diathesis Haemorrhagica 29: 228–239
39. ICTH/ICSH 1979 Prothrombin time standardization: report of the expert panel on oral anticoagulant control. Thrombosis and Haemostasis 42: 1073–1114
40. Kirkwood T B L (personal communication)
41. Langdell R D, Wagner R H, Brinkhous K M 1953 Effect of antihemophilic factor on one-stage clotting tests. A presumptive test for hemophilia and a simple one-stage

antihemophilic factor assay procedure. Journal of Laboratory and Clinical Medicine 41: 637–647
42. Bell W N, Alton H G 1954 A brain extract as a substitute for platelet suspensions in the thromboplastin generation test. Nature 174: 880–881
43. Waaler B A 1959 Contact activation in the intrinsic blood clotting system. Scandinavian Journal of Clinical and Laboratory Investigation Suppl 11: 37–44
44. Proctor R R, Rapaport S I 1961 The partial thromboplastin time with kaolin. American Journal of Clinical Pathology 36: 212–219
45. Soloway H B, Belliveau R R, Grayson J W Jr, Butler J J 1972 The in vitro effect of heparin on the partial thromboplastin time. American Journal of Clinical Pathology 58: 405–407
46. Shapiro G A, Huntzinger S W, Wilson J E 1977 Variations among commercial activated partial thromboplastin time reagents in response to heparin. American Journal of Clinical Pathology 67: 477–480
47. Sibley C S, Singer J W, Wood R T 1973 Comparison of activated partial thromboplastin reagents. American Journal of Clinical Pathology 59: 581–586
48. Hofmann J J M L, Meulendijk P N 1978 Comparison of reagents for determining the activated partial thromboplastin time. Thrombosis and Haemostasis 39: 640–645
49. Babson A L, Babson S R 1974 Comparative evaluation of a partial thromboplastin reagent containing a non-settling particulate activator. American Journal of Clinical Pathology 62: 856–860
50. Barrowcliffe T W, Gray E Studies of phospholipid reagents used in coagulation. I: Some general properties and their sensitivity to Factor VIII Thrombosis and Haemostasis: in press
51. Barrowcliffe T W, Gray E Studies of phospholipid reagents used in coagulation. II: Factors influencing their sensitivity to heparin Thrombosis and Haemostasis: in press
52. Lenahan J G, Phillips G E 1966 Some variables which influence the activated partial thromboplastin time assay. Clinical Chemistry 12: 269–273
53. Hardisty R M, Hutton R A 1965 The kaolin clotting time of platelet rich plasma — a test of platelet factor 3 availability. British Journal of Haematology 11: 258–268
54. Poller L, Thomson J M 1972 The partial thromboplastin (cephalin) time test. Journal of Clinical Pathology 25: 1038–1044
55. Denson K W E 1976 The preparation of general reagents and coagulation factors. In: Biggs R (ed) Human blood coagulation, haemostasis and thrombosis. Blackwell, Oxford, Appendix I, p 657–659
56. Giddings J C 1980 Hereditary coagulation disorders: laboratory techniques. In: Thomson J M (ed) Blood coagulation and haemostasis: a practical guide. Churchill Livingstone, Edinburgh, ch 4, p 117–157
57. Ratnoff O D, Crum J D 1964 Activation of Hageman factor by solutions of ellagic acid. Journal of Laboratory and Clinical Medicine 63: 359–377
58. Hathaway W E, Assmus S L, Montgomery R R, Dubansky A S 1979 Activated partial thromboplastin time and minor coagulopathies. American Journal of Clinical Pathology 71: 22–25
59. Poller L, Thomson J M, Yee K F 1980 Heparin and partial thromboplastin time: an international survey. British Journal of Haematology 44: 161–165
60. Janson T, Grimmer Ø 1976 Test conditions and sensitivity of the activated partial thromboplastin time (APTT) test 'Cephotest'. Saertrykk av Farmkoterapi 32: 36–46
61. Biggs R, Macfarlane R G 1962 Human blood coagulation and its disorders. Blackwell, Oxford, ch 5, p 67–85
62. Marcus A J 1966 The role of lipids in blood coagulation. Advances in Lipid Research 4: 1–37
63. Barrowcliffe T W, Stocks J, Gray E 1981 Preparation of a stable phospholipid reagent for coagulation assays. Haemostasis (in press)
64. Barrowcliffe T W, Gutteridge J M C, Dormandy T L 1975 The effect of fatty acid autoxidation products on blood coagulation. Thrombosis et Diathesis Haemorrhagica 33: 271–277
65. Poller L, Thomson J M, Palmer M K 1975 Measuring partial thromboplastin time — an assessment of the performance in serial studies. Journal of Clinical Pathology 35: 251
66. Poller L, Thomson J M, Palmer M K 1976 Measuring partial thromboplastin time. An international collaborative study. Lancet 1: 842–846
67. Triplett D A, Harms C S, Koepke J A 1978 The effect of heparin on the activated partial thromboplastin time. American Journal of Clinical Pathology 70: 556–559
68. Ingram G I C, North W R S 1981 The diagnosis of mild haemophilia by the partial thromboplastin time test. WFH/ICTH study of the Manchester method. Thrombosis and Haemostosis, 45: 162–168

69. Basu D, Gallus A, Hirsh J 1972 A prospective study of the value of monitoring heparin treatment with the activated partial thromboplastin time. New England Journal of Medicine 287: 324–327
70. Hirsh J, Gallus A S 1973 The activated partial thromboplastin time. New England Journal of Medicine 288: 1410
71. Hattersley P G 1979 Heparin and the activated partial thromboplastin time. American Journal of Clinical Pathology (letter) 71: 480
72. Triplett D A, Harms C S, Koepke J 1979. American Journal of Clinical Pathology (letter) 71: 480–481
73. Thomas D P 1978 Heparin in the prophylaxis and treatment of venous thrombosis. Seminars in Haematology 15: 1–17
74. Wessler S, Gitel S N 1979 Heparin: new concepts relevant to clinical use. Blood 53: 525–544
75. Meade T W, North W R S 1977 Population-based distributions of haemostatic variables. British Medical Bulletin 33: 283–288
76. Barrowcliffe T W, Kirkwood T B L 1981 Principles of bioassays of haemostatic components. In: Bloom A L, Thomas D P (eds) Haemostasis and thrombosis. Churchill Livingstone, Edinburgh, ch 50, 832–844
77. Kirkwood T B L, Snape T J 1980 Biometric principles in clotting and clot lysis assays. Clinical and Laboratory Haematology 2: 155–167
78. Haemophilia Centre Directors' Working Party on Standardization of Factor VIII Assay 1981 A survey of VIII:C assay in the United Kingdom. Clinical and Laboratory Haematology 3: 186–189
79. Bangham D R, Biggs R, Brozovic M, Denson K W E, Skegg J L 1971 A biological standard for measurement of blood coagulation factor VIII activity. Bulletin of the World Health Organization 45: 337–351
80. World Health Organization 1971 Technical Reports Series 463: 14
81. Barrowcliffe T W, Kirkwood T B L 1978 An international collaborative assay of Factor VIII clotting activity. Thrombosis and Haemostasis 40: 260–271
82. World Health Organization 1977 Technical Report Series 610: 12–13
83. Kirkwood T B L, Barrowcliffe T W 1978 Discrepancy between one-stage and two-stage assay of Factor VIII:C. British Journal of Haematology 40: 333–338
84. Bangham D R, Brozovic M 1974 Factor VIII International Units and reference materials. Thrombosis et Diathesis Haemorrhagica 31: 3–11
85. World Health Organization 1982 Technical Report Series (to be published)
86. Barrowcliffe T W 1981 A stable international reference plasma for Factor VIII related activities. Report of ICTH subcommittee on Factor VIII, Toronto
87. Kirkwood T B L, Rizza C R, Snape T J, Rhymes I L, Austen D E C 1977 Identification of sources of inter-laboratory variation in Factor VIII assay. British Journal of Haematology 37: 559–568
88. Barrowcliffe T W, Kemball-Cook G 1981 Modifications to the two-stage assay of Factor VIII (to be published)
89. Barrowcliffe T W, Kirkwood T B L, Rizza C R 1980 Aluminium hydroxide adsorption and Factor VIII clotting assays. Lancet 1: 820
90. Nilsson I M, Kirkwood T B L, Barrowcliffe T W 1979 In vivo recovery of Factor VIII: a comparison of one-stage and two-stage assay methods. Thrombosis and Haemostasis 42: 1230–1239
91. Harms C S, Triplett D A, Koepke J A 1978 Factor VIII (antihaemophilic factor) assay results in the 1976 College of American Pathologists survey program. American Journal of Clinical Pathology 70: Suppl 560–562
92. Brozovic M, Robertson I, Kirkwood T B L 1976 Study of a proposed international standard for blood coagulation factor IX. Thrombosis and Haemostasis 35: 222–236
93. World Health Organization 1977 Technical Report Series 610: 13
94. Barrowcliffe T W, Tydeman M S, Kirkwood T B L 1979 Major effect of prediluent in Factor IX clotting assay. Lancet 2: 192
95. Ratnoff O D, Menzie A B 1951 A new method for the determination of plasma fibrinogen in small samples of plasma. Journal of Laboratory and Clinical Medicine 37: 316–320
96. Koepke J A 1978 An innovative method for the determination of normal values in hematology using peer group laboratories. American Journal of Clinical Pathology 70, Suppl 577–579
97. Robertson I, Gaffney P J, Bangham D R 1975 Standard for human thrombin. Thrombosis et Diathesis Haemorrhagica 34: 3–19
98. Barrowcliffe T W, Johnson E A, Thomas D P 1978 Antithrombin III and heparin. British Medical Bulletin 34: 143–150

99. Kirkwood T B L, Barrowcliffe T W, Thomas D P 1980 An international collaborative study establishing a reference preparation for antithrombin III. Thrombosis and Haemostasis 43: 10–15
100. Yin E T, Wessler S, Butler J V 1973 Plasma heparin: a unique practical, submicrogram-sensitive assay. Journal of Laboratory and Clinical Medicine 81: 298–310
101. Denson K W E, Bonnar J 1973 The measurement of heparin. A method based on the potentiation of anti-factor Xa. Thrombosis et Diathesis Haemorrhagica 30: 471–479
102. Michalski R, Lane D A, Pepper D S, Kakkar V V 1978 Neutralization of heparin in plasma by platelet factor 4 and protamine sulphate. British Journal of Haematology 38: 561–571

5
Quality Control of Batch Assays
J. S. L. Fowler

INTRODUCTION

Possession of evidence assuring quality of work is of twofold importance: firstly to the laboratory, providing confidence and justifiable pride in data released; secondly to the user, that is the pathologist or clinician and hence ultimately to the patient. The users of data are usually not expert in the technical aspects of the work of the laboratory: to enable full benefit to be realized from clinical laboratory data the users must have complete confidence in the accuracy (i.e. truth) and precision (i.e. repeatability) of the laboratory's results.

We are well used to fulfilling these expectations with respect to the usual parameters and the use of automated blood counting equipment has contributed greatly to these ends. With respect to cell differentiation and morphology high quality work has been ensured by devotion of painstaking and meticulous effort: whilst this is unlikely to change in the near future, some of the automated cell differentiation equipment is beginning to provide good results. Added advantages are that this approach leads to good reproducibility and by retaining coordinates of unclassified cells can be used to enable second opinions to be sought from colleagues or consultants. Therefore, with the commonly measured parameters there are good grounds for optimism regarding quality of data, and we should expect and demand the confidence that we deserve from users. Whenever an unexpected result arises then confirmation of that value should be sought immediately. This is usually achieved by repeating the determination but if this is not possible then the probability of that result being incorrect is assessed by reference to other data obtained at about the same time. The possibility that an unexpected result is in fact a wrong result should not enter the users mind, or at least be low on his list of alternatives: it should, however, be higher on our own list.

Samples intended for the assay of parameters which are not part of the usual hour-by-hour workload must be carefully set aside and stored until the laboratory is ready to handle them. The gathering together of such samples is the batching process and the assay of these is the 'batch assay'. Batched samples in hematology are often stored as plasma or serum and are designated for assays such as folate, iron, Vitamin B_{12} or ferritin. The control of the quality of a laboratory service must encompass all aspects of the laboratories activities. With intermittent batch assays some of the problems assume particular importance. It is these aspects which will be discussed first.

The decision to set aside and periodically assay samples for certain parameters should not be taken lightly. For example, it might be better to pass such samples onto another laboratory which is in a better position to handle the work: there is no virtue in offering a wide range of assays if quality and cost-effectiveness cannot be guaranteed. Batch assays may well require the competent operation of a variety of equipment not normally encountered in day-to-day work. Additionally, there is likely to be a requirement for different reagents, calibration and control materials.

If the decision to do some assays on a periodic basis is taken then a clear policy should be established regarding who shall do them. They could be regarded as an irksome additional chore to be undertaken at the end of the week by someone with spare time or alternatively they could be regarded as a challenging task which can be undertaken by specifically experienced people who have been given the necessary training and resources to achieve a good performance.

Individuals who intend to work on batch assays should be widely trained and experienced. They should have become experienced under supervision and must have demonstrated an ability to work independently to a very high standard before being expected to report results from patient specimens. If the laboratory is unable or unwilling to spare commitment from such well qualified personnel then the decision to undertake the unusual non-routine work should be reviewed and, preferably, the specimens should be referred to another laboratory. Of course, such decisions are rarely completely clear-cut and very satisfactory arrangements can be made whereby neighbouring laboratories specialize in one or other technique, thus, in effect, pooling their resources. The overriding factors of all such decisions of whether, where and who shall do a particular assay must of course be ultimately related to provision of maximum benefit to the patient.

KEY FEATURES OF GOOD PERFORMANCE IN BATCH ASSAYS

In our laboratories three maxims are observed: quality, turnround and 'customer' satisfaction. These are of general importance, but they may create particular difficulties in batch assays. The laboratory which consistently provides high quality data is immediately identifiable as possessing high morale internally, and externally is regarded with respect; good quality must also be accompanied by good turnround of results but this may be difficult to achieve with batched samples. Customer satisfaction is based on attainment of quality and turnround objectives: however, it also depends on other less definable factors, one of which is provision of a range of relevant and proven techniques appropriate to the clinicians' needs and patient population. This is not to be taken as an obligation to provide a service which is purely reactive to the clinicians'/patients' perceived needs: it is essential that the hematology laboratory utilizes all its powers of advocacy and diplomacy in promoting interest in useful methods and diminishing interest in less helpful techniques. Neither must the laboratory confuse 'useful method' with 'easy to do method' or 'unhelpful method' with 'difficult to do method'. It is far better to master a few really useful techniques and devote resources to these than to try and offer an overwide service.

STANDARD PROTOCOL FOR BATCH ASSAY METHODS

In industrial laboratories over the years the practice has developed of preparing documentation relating to each method. Recently this has been formalized in response to government guidelines, in particular the American guidelines issued by the Food and Drug Administration (FDA)[1] and Environmental Protection Agency (EPA),[2] and has led to the standard operating procedure (SOP).

Although the Americans have been in the forefront with good laboratory and good manufacturing practice (GLP and GMP) there are signs that most governments are moving along similar lines. The scope of government influence also appears to be steadily increasing, although local changes may occasionally slow this down. As well as GLP and GMP, it seems possible that good clinical practice (GCP) guidelines may eventually influence the clinical laboratory.

The standard operating procedure (SOP) concept can be of value in many parts of the laboratory, and not only in documentation of methods. SOPs should be prepared to define all activities of the laboratory including the processes of sample reception, separation, storage (particularly important for batched assays), identification and eventual disposal. The SOP can be seen as fulfilling a need not catered for by the scientific journals or manufacturers' literature: an SOP should be prepared as a detailed description of exactly how to do a job in your own laboratory under your conditions (Fig. 5.1). SOPs must be kept up to date and must be freely available at the bench. Their role may be seen as providing: a checklist for experienced personnel; a training aid for inexperienced personnel; and a historical record of methods. SOPs may also acquire increased medico-legal significance in the litigious future.

Use of and adherence to an SOP policy will avoid the problem of unintentional, or even intentional, modification of methods. It is often not sufficient to simply refer to a published method because its local application will require some minor modification and it is important to keep records of such alterations.

Fig. 5.1 Layout of a standard operating procedure (SOP).

CLINICAL TOXICOLOGY STANDARD OPERATING PROCEDURE	REF NO ★	★ Amendment code e.g. 1st method: 00 revised method: 01 2nd revision: 02 etc
To boil water: electric kettle method *Work Routine*: 1. Fill kettle so that element is covered. 2. Replace lid with vent directed away. 3. Plug into socket and switch on. 4. Switch off when steam issues freely. 5. Remove plug from socket. 6. Pour water taking care to avoid steam or splashing. 7. Pour any residual water to waste to minimize scaling. 8. Place kettle in a safe place to cool.		*Amendment Procedure* To amend a method, the outdated SOP should be overstamped "AMENDED", initialled and dated then archived in a historical file. The revised method will be allocated the same reference number but with a suffix (as above): and the new signatures will be overstamped "AMENDMENT".
Signatures: (authorized Scientific Officer) Date: (Supervisor)		

This is particularly important in large laboratories with specialized subdivisions which need to be aware of the implications of change on other parts of the service. When continuous modifications are made to even the simplest method it may often be difficult for staff who normally work in other areas to step into the breach adequately in an emergency without the appropriate SOP. In order to maintain quality of results all method details must be recorded, since it is only when things go wrong that apparently minor procedural deviations can be evaluated regarding their contribution to the observed error.

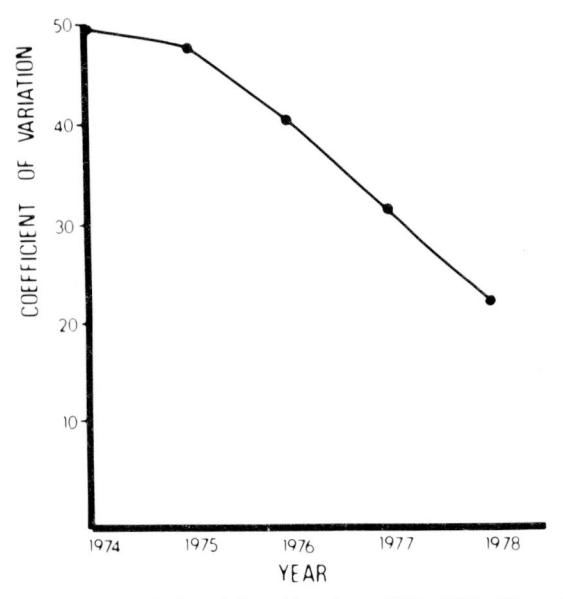

Fig.5.2 Trend in coefficient of variation, folic acid analysis, 1974–1978. (From Hansell & Haven, 1979.[3])

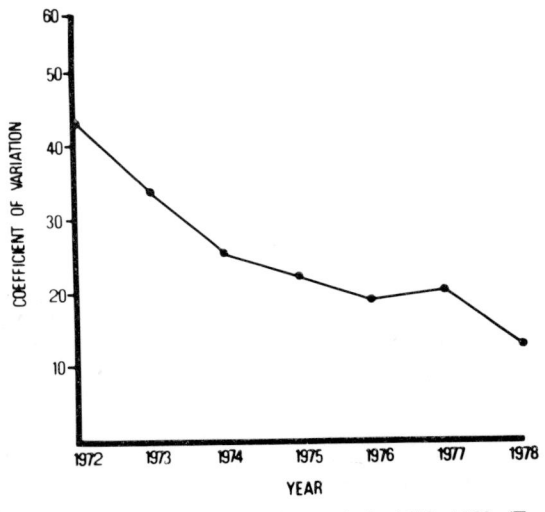

Fig. 5.3 Trend in coefficient of variation, vitamin B_{12} analysis, 1972–1978. (From Hansell & Haven, 1979.[3])

In summary, unwritten rules and word of mouth modifications are inconsistent with quality control and should not be tolerated in the laboratory. Historical files containing outdated SOPs can illustrate the evolution of method details: these can be helpful when studying trends in laboratory performance year-by-year (Figs. 5.2 and 5.3).

CHOICE OF METHODS FOR BATCH ASSAYS

The major contributions to error in a result for a patient's sample, as opposed to a control, arise from combinations of the following:

1. Laboratory components of error
a. Taking the sample.
b. Choice of container, diluent, anticoagulant.
c. Labeling the sample.
d. Transporting the sample.
e. Receiving and separating the sample.
f. Storage of the sample.
g. Aliquoting the sample.
h. Analyzing the sample.
i. Recording the result.
j. Transmitting the result.
k. Interpreting the result.
l. Action arising from the interpretation.

2. Physiological components of error
a. In the individual, due to inadequate preparation — for example fasting/non-fasting.
b. In the individual, due to stress of surroundings or sampling technique.
c. In the individual, due to interference by concomitant therapy.
d. In the individual, due to simultaneous investigation by other diagnostic techniques.

In this section, which relates to choice of methods for batch assays, discussion centres mainly on point 1 (h). The list puts this in its wider context. Failure in any one item could negate the whole exercise.

Great care is warranted in the choice of method itself. If a laboratory is to go to the trouble of storing samples for, let us say, a weekly run of a particular methodology, with all the consequent problems of stability of the constituent and maintenance of sample identification, then it makes sense to employ the most reliable method of analysis.

It is important that every new method considered for the clinical laboratory should undergo evaluation in the laboratory in which it is to be used. Even before the evaluation begins, a search of the literature for evidence of satisfactory performance, including the accuracy, precision, and specificity of the method is desirable: to study a method properly we must examine the written protocol which should give in detail the steps the analyst must follow. Ideally, preliminary runs should be made with calibrators and a few samples of a pooled reference material to develop familiarity with the procedure. At this stage, substantial problems relating to reproducibility, sensitivity, linearity, analytical noise, and instrument adequacy may be detected. Any shortcomings should be carefully recorded and then corrected, or the method may be rejected with a minimum expenditure of effort. It is important to record all problems encountered even at this stage since such findings may form the basis for preventative maintenance schedules at a later date. If the method being considered for batch use is not rejected in such a preliminary study, precision should be assessed by repeatedly analyzing a number of aliquots of pooled samples which embrace as wide a range of concentrations as possible, relevant to likely patient samples. Reference materials should be used if they are available. This can be followed by a program of analysis which contains replicate patient samples, randomly allocated. Means and standard deviations can then be calculated for each of the materials and the component of error due to laboratory causes can be compared with that due to physiological causes. It may be that a method is clinically useful even when it is not inherently very precise.[4] This can be so, especially if the analyte shows a wide variation in the body in disease (Table 5.1).

It can easily be seen that automation of certain methods such as calcium and hemoglobin should receive higher priority than those for bilirubin or sodium. The relatively poor precision of the bilirubin method is tolerable since quite large changes will occur in disease and these will be recognizable despite methodological 'noise'.

Finally, some measure of long-range reproducibility should be made before a method is accepted and used: to achieve this, analytical runs should be carried out with new sets of reagents on different days and, if feasible, with different laboratory staff. It is not unusual for a method that appears good at the beginning to fail under extended testing of this type.

Table 5.1 Comparison of critical coefficient of variation (CV) for various parameters with analytical precision of their measurement.

Parameter	Level	Critical CV*	Mean CV Manual	Mean CV Automated
Calcium	11.0 mg/dl	2.27	3.09	2.12
Sodium	150 mEq/ℓ	1.33	1.10	1.04
Osmolality	270 mOsm/kg	1.7	1.75	—
Hemoglobin	10 g/dl	4.0	4.78	3.35
Bilirubin	1 mg/dl	20.0	12.48	7.77
	6 mg/dl		5.27	3.76

$$CV = \text{coefficient of variation} = \frac{SD \times 100}{\text{mean}}$$

*Critical CV = medically significant CV (after Ross & Fraser, 1979)[4]

ASSESSMENT OF ACCURACY OF A METHOD

It may be possible to arrange for selected samples which have been used to measure the precision of a method to be analyzed by a reference method or other procedure of known high quality, in order to establish the accuracy (or lack of it) in that method. Once again, patient samples encompassing the usable concentration range should be analyzed by both methods to establish correlation and repeatability over the method's range.

Although not strictly relevant to batch methods used in hematology it is interesting to note that recovery experiments are an essential part of the evaluation of most chemical methods especially in the absence of a reference method. In this approach, known amounts of pure analyte are added to a previously analyzed sample, usually in two or three increments. Aliquots of these specimens are tested to determine the recovery of added analyte: the amount of analyte recovered should be within ±5 per cent of the amount added. Low recovery indicates poor specificity, inadequate calibration, or just a plain bad method. This approach would not be easily applicable in the case of say folate, iron or ferritin assays where there may be doubt in establishing the appropriate pure analyte to be added or difficulty in mimicking its physiological form.

If adequate studies were not conducted and reported by the authors of the method, investigations for specificity must be initiated before the method is put into routine practice.[5] The laboratory should never accept the assurance of others. Common, potentially interfering substances should be added to previously analyzed patient specimens at levels that may be encountered clinically. For example, if special drugs are a part of the treatment for patients for whom this test is to be performed, then the effects of the presence of these drugs and their metabolites if any, should be determined. If a substance is found to cause interference in a particular method then the laboratory is faced with several alternatives. It may be necessary not to use the method when that substance is present, to remove the substance before the method is used, or to determine the amount of interference separately. If these alternatives are not practical and interference is suspected, then a more specific method must be found.

In the absence of a reference method, and if commercial reference materials are available with assigned values which have been arrived at using well accepted techniques, then these may afford the most practical basis for evaluating the accuracy of a test method. In practice, it may be desirable to use more than one batch of reference material and preferably batches from several different sources. Reference materials should be analyzed a sufficient number of times to give a statistically valid comparison with which to establish the bias of the candidate method values in relation to the reference material value.

INTERLABORATORY EXCHANGE SCHEMES

Participation in interlaboratory comparisons and proficiency testing programs involving common reference materials or patient specimens, affords further opportunities to evaluate analytical bias. It is often assumed that the true results will be close to the mean from all laboratories using the same method. Although such an assumption is somewhat sweeping, repeated discrepancies may provide a warning that special accuracy studies are needed.

There are two main types of quality control program commonly used in clinical laboratories. Intralaboratory procedures are essential in every laboratory and must be entirely internal, although they may involve some external data processing service. Interlaboratory programs provide an entirely blind system of external quality control which when grafted onto an adequate internal program can give the following advantages:[6]
1. An independent assessment of laboratory performance.
2. A comparison of analytical accuracy to encourage convergence of data in all parts of the world.
3. Greater interest in 'state-of-the-art' performance.

Taken together these advantages will lead to the build up of independent information concerning the precision and accuracy of the different methods that are used by the participants.

A typical interlaboratory program is organized on a six-monthly cycle. Before the start of each cycle, participants are asked to complete a questionnaire concerning their assay methods and other relevant laboratory variables. A kit of materials sufficient for the complete cycle is then supplied. Such a kit might contain a set of 12 dated samples in duplicate which are to be assayed one every two weeks together with cards on which to enter the assay results, addressed return envelopes for the results cards, progress charts and full operating instructions. Each sample for assay would probably consist of two bottles of freeze-dried serum and every two weeks during the six-month cycle, tests are carried out on the appropriate sample, the assays being performed as and when the laboratory schedule permits but with the aim of posting the results to arrive in time for the target date for computer processing. This approach will enable the laboratory to contribute to the consensus view regarding a particular value attributed to the sample.

USE OF REFERENCE RANGES FROM OTHER LABORATORIES

It is important to be aware of the values which other laboratories or textbooks regard as the 'normal range'. The word normal is, however, potentially misleading and a better choice would be 'expected range' or 'reference range'. This is because these values incorporate variability from several sources not only from the patients, but also from the laboratory. Ranges of reference values must therefore be determined or verified by each clinical laboratory. Substantial disagreements with the ranges published by other laboratories that use the same method could serve to warn of possible bias. On the other hand, agreement may be used as justification for acceptance of a published reference range without need for further extensive studies of healthy populations. Laboratory and hospital personnel who claim to be in good health may themselves provide a useful study population to supplement other accuracy investigations. However, this approach must only be adopted with great care since it is likely that these groups are younger and more active than the patient population and this difference may well be reflected in the values for the parameter being considered. If, having taken into account these possible pitfalls, it can be established that the mean of a fairly normal population is similar to the mean of the published reference range, then equivalent calibration (i.e. accuracy) may be inferred.

STATISTICAL APPROACH TO METHOD EVALUATION

A number of statistical tests may be used in the evaluation of methods as long as one remembers that statistical calculations do not determine acceptability but rather provide estimates of the type and magnitude of error. Sufficient method evaluation data should be gathered to provide bias and imprecision estimates at a variety of relevant concentration levels so that a regression analysis can be carried out. As a part of the evaluation, test results versus reference method results should be plotted on a graph that also portrays a least squares estimate of the line representing their relationship. The slope, intercept, extent of correlation and reasons for and magnitude of deviations from this regression line should be considered (see Appendix: Simple Statistics, p. 182).

When the evaluation of a method has been completed, precision and accuracy will have been estimated for the concentration range over which it is to be used. The decision to keep, reject or possibly modify the method on the basis of this information as well as other factors that may be peculiar to the laboratory (costs, sensitivity, efficiency of time and materials, space, equipment, level of difficulty of execution of the procedure, and safety considerations) can now be taken.

Method evaluation continues for as long as the method is in use. The ongoing evaluation should consist of inspection of control charts and other records such as log books for indications of poor performance. Special long-range control charts on which the means of control results for each week or month are plotted, may be used to detect trends and shifts that are not easily seen in short-range charts. The cusum methods for analyzing such control data are discussed in Chapters 1 and 6.

Performance should be reviewed and discussed openly by the laboratory team on a regular (weekly or monthly) basis since ultimately control of quality depends on successful collaboration between people and not on possession of mountains of control charts or reference materials and printouts. The people referred to in this concept are of course primarily the laboratory analysts but also must include the suppliers of various materials, clinicians, nurses, laboratory aides, the list is potentially a long one. Points arising in discussions between analysts should be recorded and added to a method record; this record could be regarded as a log book for the method.

Log books

It has proved very well worthwhile to keep a record by each instrument of when it was used and by whom, together with details of regular maintenance and problems which are encountered. This approach is particularly appropriate for laboratories faced with the problem of batch assays. It is, for example, vital to ensure regular maintenance of batch assay equipment even if its use appears to be sporadic. There is no reason why an instrument log book concept could not be extended to become a method log book. In this case it would form part of the basis for the regular laboratory discussions referred to above. In our own laboratory the quality control officer keeps a quality control log book, which together with the instrument logbooks, fulfills this purpose. The ongoing method evaluation which is possible on the basis of this logged information also leads to a program of preventative maintenance. Although this may appear expensive in terms of service contracts and time, it will go a long way to ensuring that poor data is neither generated or released from the laboratory. It is all part of the laboratory's control of quality.

Methods going 'out of control'
Ongoing method evaluation may reveal chronic problems that need corrective action which may be only indirectly related to the method itself. For example, imprecision that regularly exceeds performance criteria may often be reduced with the help of special training to improve skills and techniques of laboratory staff. Alternatively, the solution may be in substituting more automated volumetric equipment for manual pipettes or simply by better equipment usage and maintenance.

Excessive bias may also appear in a previously acceptable method. This fault may be often traced to changes in methodology or equipment, miscalibrated equipment, or deterioration in calibrators or reagents. Although correction usually is simple, diagnosis may be difficult. Of course, prompt efficient diagnosis of any problem is facilitated by adequate laboratory records (for example the log books). Reserve supplies of tested standard and reagent solutions may be particularly helpful in the diagnostic process enabling detection of deteriorating materials.

To summarize what can be done with methods to ensure high quality of batch assay performance, the following check list may be helpful:
1. Decide which assays to do and which to refer to other laboratories.
2. Decide if facilities are adequate for the chosen assays.
3. Prepare standard-operating procedures for the chosen assays and use log books.
4. Identify the major sources of foreseeable error for each method.
5. Assess the method in your own laboratory.
6. Develop an internal quality control system.
7. Collaborate in an interlaboratory quality control scheme.
8. Develop an on-going evaluative approach with corresponding preventative maintenance.

Finally, when any amendments are made to a method, the entire method should be studied again for precision, accuracy and specificity.

A change in method may appear simple and yet it may be responsible for increased susceptibility to an interference that was not present before, a decrease in precision, an increased bias, or other difficulties in performance. If any method change is implemented then it must be documented in the standard operating procedure with a dated entry in the log book.

Using the method
Care in selection of methods must be accompanied by correct use of reagents, instruments and reference materials if high quality data is to be produced.

Reagents

Reagent-grade or even higher purity materials should be used and occasionally purification steps will form part of the method. If this is the case then details should be included in the SOP. Containers for reagents should be carefully labeled with the date of the receipt, and expiry if applicable, so that some form of inventory control can be established. This will help to ensure that there is always sufficient reagent available and that deteriorated materials are discarded before they spoil assay results. It is useful to record the reagent blank absorbance value in the method log book, so keeping an eye on conditions of reagents.

When standard solutions are prepared these must be calibrated with respect to primary standards. If the standard solutions have to be prepared frequently then this connection is readily made if the preparation data is recorded in the method log book. If standard solutions are prepared centrally for use by several analysts then a centralized 'standards log book' will be useful since each standard solution may be numbered and a record kept of the identity, date prepared, formulators initials and expiry date. Use of the reagent solution could then be recorded in the method log book by simply quoting the standard solution number.

Supplies of good quality water are almost always essential either as a reagent or for final rinsing of glassware: filtered deionized water or double distilled water is the most reliable. This assumes that it is carefully stored: contamination during storage[8] is a common cause of problems and it may be worthwhile to institute periodic checks of stored water if this is suspected.

Reagent kits

Kits can be a useful, if expensive, approach to handling a periodic demand for special assays. A suitable evaluation scheme applicable to a candidate reagent kit would involve repeated analysis of pooled samples and also of reference materials from a variety of sources. Estimates of precision and accuracy should be obtained over a wide range of concentrations representative of those likely to be encountered in use. If the kit method is a replacement for an existing approach then a careful comparison of the two methods should be made by correlating results from patient samples analyzed in duplicate over a wide range of values. If the laboratory intending to use the kit has no relevant experience on which to base such an evaluation, then patient samples can be exchanged and simultaneously analyzed by an experienced centre prepared to act as reference laboratory. Purchase of a kit implies acquisition of method expertise, high quality reagents and reliable reference materials: this is why they are expensive. Making use of kits requires a considerable act of faith in the manufacturers, it is to be hoped that they give value for money.

Instruments

Instrument policy is very influential with respect to quality of results. There is a wide choice of manual or automated instruments and consequently a need to choose, operate and maintain such equipment in such a manner as to avoid generation of poor quality data.

Instrument performance can be assessed retrospectively in terms of results from patient or quality control program samples. Satisfactory results from retrospective surveys provide re-assurance, but contribute less than prospective checks. Application of prospective checks can lead to a high degree of control which can anticipate the onset of problems before they become observable in results and certainly before they are of any consequence in differential diagnosis of clinical disease. In day-to-day terms, it obviously contributes to efficiency if it can be noted that an instrument is not performing correctly prior to commitment of patient samples. This is particularly important in batched assays where the opportunity to obtain repeat samples is limited or absent. We all know that problems stemming from generation of poor results can be be considerably more time consuming than the measures that would have been needed to avoid generating these results in the first place.

Non-automated instruments

Spectrophotometric or colorimetric instruments are particularly susceptible to electrical interferences and poor siting. Electrical variations such as voltage fluctuation or interference from nearby equipment can lead to apparently random variation in display or readouts. Careful screening of spectrophotometric equipment and use of stabilized power sources will usually overcome these electrical problems.

A second problem which may be encountered is due to poor positioning, for example, on a bench receiving direct sunlight. Cuvette housings usually have a matt black finish and this can lead to high internal temperatures, especially in direct sunlight. Problems can also arise from poorly fitting or incompletely baffled cuvette compartment covers which allow entry of stray light. Sunlight in particular can vary in intensity rapidly during determination of a batch of samples, leading to variable and puzzling results.

Care in selection and siting of even the simplest instruments will pay dividends by improving quality of results. Assuming that a stable power supply and environment are available then care must be taken when setting up the instrument for each batch of assays. A useful prospective check for variable wavelength spectrophotometers is to check the settings of monochromators by use of reference materials before batches of patient samples are committed. Potassium dichromate (340 nm) or cobalt acetate (540 nm) stock solutions or internal standards such as a didymium filter can be employed to provide assurance of correct function.

Automated instruments

In general an increase in precision is obtained by transferring from a good manual to a good automated method (Fig. 5.1). Often, good results can be obtained with a variety of analytical methods although as usual of course it is those with which we are most experienced which seem most satisfactory. Usually it will be cost-effective to use automated (not automatic) methodologies since more work can be done in a given time and more consistent results obtained. Sample volume and reagent savings frequently result from adoption of automated methodologies. Such factors can be important in batch processing and should enable attainment of high precision with optimal use of quality control materials.

'Automated' methodologies help to take some drudgery out of laboratory life and should not be confused with so-called 'automatic' methods. In this concept there is little involvement of staff and this almost invariably leads to a poor quality of results. It must never be inferred that people have little to do with the quality of results, since this is never the case. Another important aspect of the automated approach to analysis is that usually data acquisition systems are available with such instruments; these will minimize manual data transcription which is a notorious source of error.

Automated instruments are conveniently classified into two types: continuous-flow (Technicon-type) or discrete analyzers. The discrete systems are more important in handling the batch assays of the hematology laboratory. Discrete analytical systems consist of sampling, reagent addition, incubation, photometric and readout functions which are fully integrated in the most completely automated systems. Monitoring the performance of these analytical systems is complex, since often the various functions are interrelated in some way. The use of manufacturers quality control materials, monitoring devices and dial settings is usually insufficient. In any case, at the outset prior to purchase preferably or at least on purchase of the instrument, the manufacturers claims for sampling precision, equilibration times, temperatures, spectrophotometer performance should be scrupulously checked by use of independent instrumentation or by use of reference materials. It is also worth remembering that with imported equipment, it is as well to establish that the transformed voltages are as specified and that sufficient current is available from the transformer when connection is made to the local power supply. Apart from the function checks which must be repeated periodically, performance checks are vital on a regular basis.

Performance tests for instruments
Regular analysis of about 20 aliquots of normal and abnormal pooled patient samples should be undertaken. Data should analyzed to give the mean, range and co-efficient of variation, both in units of measurement and also in absorbance values if spectrophotometric modules are incorporated. This will provide an assessment of both attained precision and accuracy for comparison with previous performance. Good performance in absorbance checks and in terms of precision indicates that further investigation is probably not justified. A careful ongoing program of performance testing when combined with incorporation of reference material in each batch of unknowns analyzed, should provide satisfactory reassurance that a method is in control. In this respect automated and non-automated methodology do not differ, for in the hands of expert staff, either should lead to excellent results.

The use of control materials
A control material, if it is to be used for calibration should be regarded as hav-

ing two components: the analyte and the matrix. The matrix forms the bulk of control materials and since these are usually derived from biological samples then this matrix is invariably proteinaceous. This is important in that proteins vary subtly from species-to-species and also are commonly found to interfere with analyses. So it can be difficult to control data arising from patient samples if the control materials are derived from bovine or equine sources, which they often are. When employing control materials the assumption is made that their behaviour is identical with that of the patient sample in so far as the analytical process is concerned: usually ideal controls in terms of analyte and matrix will, therefore, be prepared from material of human origin. Use of these may lead to risks to human health. Interference from preservatives may also occur and care must be taken to ensure that these are not contraindicated in the analyses in question.

The storage and dispensing of control materials must not only be achieved safely but must also be controlled with great care since variation between aliquots will add greatly to imprecision of results. Control materials should always be prepared or purchased in as large batches as possible so that handover from batch to batch is as infrequent as possible. When handing over from an old to a new batch of control material a considerable degree of overlap is desirable because this enables us to maintain confidence in quality control data. Control materials are used mainly to maintain precision but control over accuracy is also essential. This can best be achieved by purchase or exchange of materials with assigned values; these should be incorporated into analytical runs as unknowns, randomly distributed into each batch of patient samples.

ATTITUDE TO QUALITY CONTROL MEASURES

Quality control measures should always be seen as a safeguard but never as a threat. The attainment of the expected values, for example, of randomly allocated samples, should be seen as a challenge, adding interest to the daily work. As stated in the introduction, the possibility that an unexpected result is in fact a wrong result should not enter the users mind. If this is the case then he is in a position to immediately act upon the data which the laboratory has produced. It is also particularly important that as far as possible, errors are avoided in batch assays since opportunities for resampling the patient or repeating the assay are unlikely to exist.

Careful choice of the method, of reagents and control materials will complete the picture ensuring that the contribution of laboratory error to the overall variability of the data is minimized: that is an important part of the laboratory's job.

REFERENCES

1. US Food and Drug Administration 1978 Non-clinical Laboratory Studies, Good Laboratory Practice Regulations 43 FR p 59986–60025
2. US Environmental Protection Agency 1979 Good Laboratory Practice for Health Effects (Proposals) 44 FR 27333–375

3. Hansell J R, Haven G T 1979 Changes in level of precision of common ligand assays during a seven-year interval. American Journal of Clinical Pathology 72 (No 2 Suppl): 320–325
4. Ross J W, Fraser M D 1979 Analytical clinical laboratory precision. American Journal of Clinical Pathology 72 (No 2 Suppl): 265–273
5. Young D S, Pestanen L C, Gibberman V 1975 Effects of drugs on clinical laboratory tests. Clinical Chemistry 21: 1D–432D
6. Wellcome Group Quality Control Programme 1981, 14th edn. Wellcome Research Laboratories, Beckenham, UK
7. Whitehead T P 1977 Quality control in clinical chemistry. Wiley, New York. ch 6, p 44–45
8. US Environmental Protection Agency, Analytical Quality Control Laboratory 1972. Handbook for analytical quality control in water and wastewater laboratories. Environmental Protection Agency. National Environmental Research Center, Analytical Quality Control Laboratory, Cincinnati

6
Standardization for Routine Blood Counting — the Role of Interlaboratory Trials
P. G. Ward   J. Wardle   S. M. Lewis

Interlaboratory trials can play an important part in maintaining laboratory proficiency. They form the basis for external quality assessment (EQA) schemes by means of which the technical skill of individual laboratories and the efficacy of their equipment can be assessed. In addition, they provide data for assessing methods for identifying the limitations and faults of a particular method, type of equipment or reagent. The most important function of an EQA scheme is to provide a means for ensuring comparability of results between laboratories. This is especially important when there is no definitive reference material available, for without an EQA scheme the individual laboratory cannot judge the comparative accuracy of its performance, even if it has a well established internal quality control system.

The College of American Pathologists (CAP) has been active in this process for about 20 years, and in the United States there are now a number of schemes organized by government agencies, e.g. Center for Disease Control (CDC), by state departments of health concerned with laboratory inspection and accreditation and by professional associations (e.g. The American Association of Bioanalysts) who are more directly interested in education rather than licensing. These schemes were, in general, initially concerned exclusively with clinical chemistry, but the need for similar control in hematology (and blood banking) was soon recognized, and the latter has become a major component in many of these services. In the past decade schemes have been organized in the United Kingdom, Canada, Australia, France, Germany and, more recently, in other countries of Western Europe, whilst the World Health Organization is promoting the development of national quality assurance programs globally. The schemes have been known by a diversity of titles, *inter alia*, Interlaboratory Quality Control, Survey Programs, Ring Testing, Proficiency Testing Program, Laboratory Improvement Program, Quality Evaluation, Interlaboratory Comparison. This diversity of terms reflects diverse purposes for such schemes. It has recently been proposed to introduce internationally agreed definitions as follows: *Internal quality control* refers to tests using reference and control materials as well as the statistical analysis of data from tests on patients' specimens, carried out within the laboratory. *External quality assessment* is the objective evaluation by an external agency, under direction of professional colleagues, of the performance by a number of laboratories on material supplied for specified tests. These two components together constitute *quality assurance*.

An EQA scheme provides specimens for interlaboratory trials and values can be assigned to these by statistical analysis of the results from all participants. This provides comparability and standardization by consensus, even if it is not possible to establish and verify the results as being absolutely true. On this basis the UK National Quality Control Scheme (now known as the UK External Quality Assessment Scheme) came into being some ten years ago.[1] This scheme has expanded to include some 500 participants, who receive material at frequent intervals, not only for blood counts, but also, less frequently, for a range of other tests, including reticulocyte counts, differential white cell counts, abnormal hemoglobins and glucose-6-phosphate dehydrogenase as well as the serum levels of vitamin B_{12}, iron, iron binding capacity, transferrin and ferritin.

PREPARATION AND STABILITY OF QUALITY CONTROL MATERIALS

As the time scale of trials prevents the use of fresh blood, various substitute preparations have been tried.[2] These include synthetic materials such as latex particles, chemically treated biological materials such as glutaraldehyde fixed cells or partly fixed blood[3] and blood which has simply been preserved. Synthetic materials and glutaraldehyde fixed blood have a virtually indefinite shelf-life with stable assigned values and constant particle size distribution. Whole blood may be preserved by collecting it into ACD (NIH-A) or CPD anticoagulant and adding an antibiotic (penicillin-streptomycin). This can be dispensed aseptically and homogeneously into a series of vials by means of a suitable mixing-dispensing unit.[4] Table 6.1 illustrates sample reproducibility with this system. Freshly collected human blood has a shelf-life of at least three weeks, whilst equine blood remains in good condition for at least three months. The UK national trials have also shown that preserved blood can be transported across the world by conventional first class air mail without appreciable deterioration. Figure 6.1 shows the relative distribution of a mixture of fixed platelets and fixed donkey red cells with clear separation between instrument noise, fixed platelet and fixed donkey cells.

Table 6.1 Reproducibility of well mixed samples of preserved whole blood.

Whole blood (2 different samples)	73 analyses on a single Coulter S system		Single analysis on 195 Coulter S systems	
	m	s	m	s
Hb (g/dl)	9.64	0.07	9.73	0.14
RBC (x 10^{12}/l)	3.18	0.02	5.43	0.12
PCV	0.294	0.002	0.286	0.010
MCV (fl)	91.42	0.50	52.67	1.97
WBC (x 10^9/l)	4.46	0.08	5.64	0.24

Fixed platelets (2 different samples)	12 analyses by manual reference method (one person)		Single analysis on 140 Coulter Thrombocounter systems	
	m	s	m	s
Platelets (x 10^9/l)	110.1	1.1	132.2	15.0

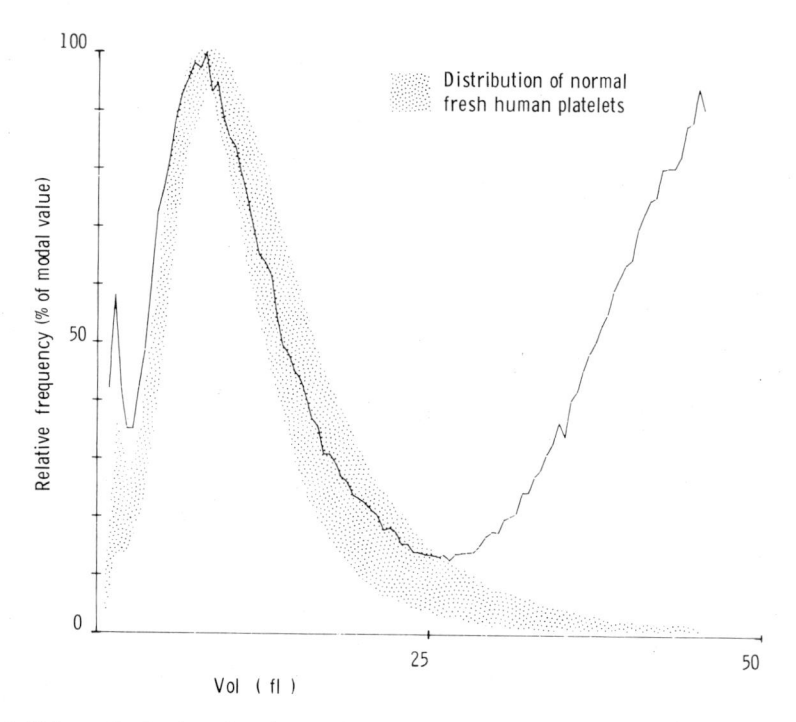

Fig. 6.1 Volume distribution of a mixture of fixed human platelets and fixed donkey red cells.

ANALYSIS OF TRIAL RESULTS

The object of the assessment is to evaluate the performance ability of individual participants and to identify problems relating to methods, instruments, reagents and control preparations in the country as a whole or in a particular region. Trial data may be analyzed by means of simple statistical computer programs.[5] In the first instance a crude mean and SD are calculated for all the data for each parameter or method for samples which arrived in laboratories the day after despatch. Values which lie outside the crude range m ± 2 SD are then excluded. Experience has shown that by this means transcription errors and poor results caused by serious errors in techniques are excluded. Values which reflect only minor disturbances are kept within the calculation. A weighted mean value and SD are then calculated from these refined data. From this, a deviation index (/R/) may be calculated for each result returned by each laboratory:

$$\text{Deviation index (/R/)} = \frac{\text{test result (x)} - \text{weighted mean (m}'\text{)}}{\text{weighted standard deviation (s}'\text{)}}$$

This index is simply a measure of how far a test result differs from the weighted mean value as a multiple of the standard deviation. Its main advantage is that it is independent of the value of the mean so that it allows accuracy for different samples and parameters to be readily compared.

To illustrate this analysis, the hemoglobin results from one group of partici-

STANDARDIZATION FOR ROUTINE BLOOD COUNTING 105

Table 6.2 Hemoglobin concentration measured by 47 laboratories using miscellaneous methods.

		Sample X	Sample Y	Ratio y/x = z
Grade A				
Crude	No	47	47	47
	Mean	12.52	9.82	0.784
	SD	0.16	0.14	0.008
	CV	1.3	1.4	1.0
Weighted	No	45	44	41
	Mean	12.53	9.82	0.783
	SD	0.14	0.11	0.006
	CV	1.0	1.1	0.7
Grade B				
Crude and weighted	No	6	6	6
	Mean	12.78	10.00	0.782
	SD	0.31	0.18	0.007
	CV	2.4	1.8	0.9

pants are presented. This group used a number of different methods and instruments. Forty-seven laboratories received their samples on the day after despatch (grade A data) and six within three days of despatch (grade B data). Table 6.2 shows the relevant crude and weighted means and standard deviations for the two samples. The x/y distribution (Youden plot) for 53 pairs of samples (Fig. 6.2), shows that most of the points are close together but that there are some outliers, and the object is to identify the reason for these. When the deviation indices for each result are plotted (Fig. 6.3) three participants can be seen to be 'poor performers' on both samples. Although /R/ does not show why the value from which it is derived was in error it does indicate that in the case of these three laboratories the error was consistent.

A further aid to understanding the cause of 'poor performance' is the ratio

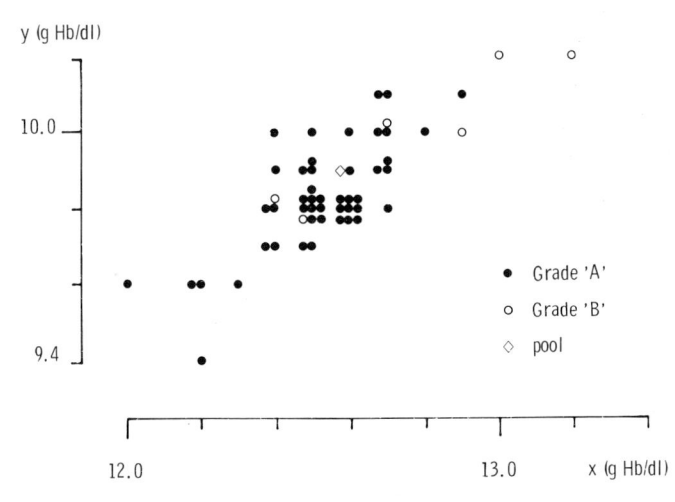

Fig. 6.2 Hemoglobin concentration for two samples (x and y) measured in 53 laboratories. 'Pool' is the mean result measured by fully automated cell counters.

106 QUALITY CONTROL

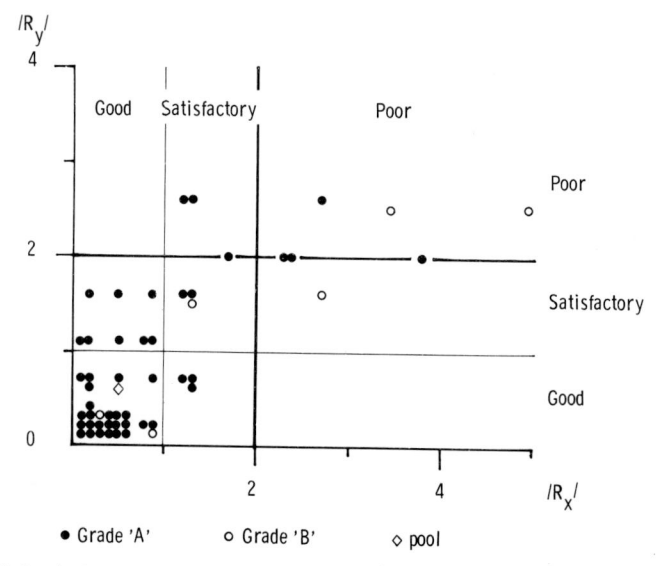

Fig. 6.3 Deviation index/R/R/ distribution for each data point in Fig. 6.2.

test. The results of this test are not printed in the UK trial reports sent to participants, but from the data supplied it is a simple matter for each laboratory to calculate the ratio z = y/x for their own results. The 'true' slope of the straight line linking the concentrations of the analyte in samples x and y is indicated by the z value for the Grade A weighted means. Figure 6.4 shows that the deviation index for the ratio ($/R_z/$) for seven laboratories were 'poor'. From this type of analysis it is possible to suggest causes for poor performance, such as incor-

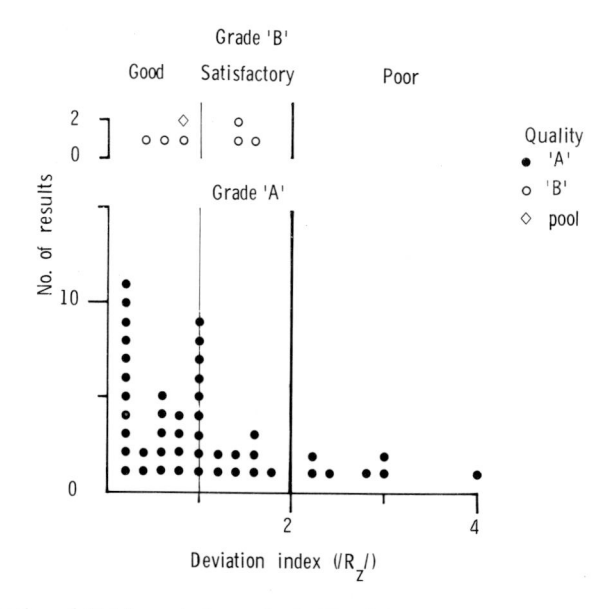

Fig. 6.4 Distribution of $/R_z/$ for each data point in Fig. 6.2.

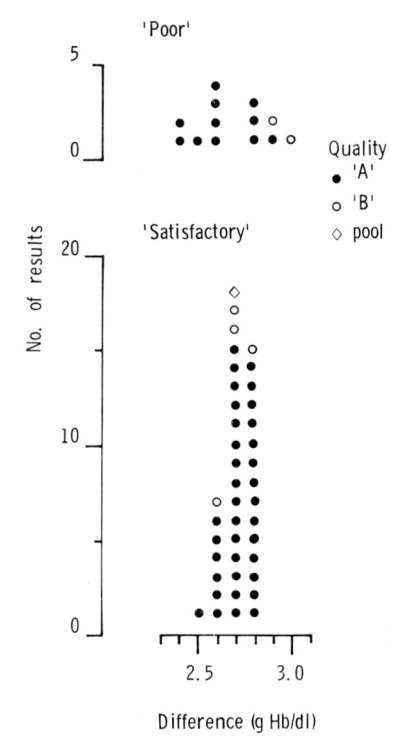

Fig. 6.5 Difference between Hb values of x and y for each data point in Fig. 6.2.

rect use of calibrator or incorrect zero setting. We have found that the difference (d) between the values of x and y (Fig. 6.5) is a further help. Table 6.3 brings together data on all the 'poor performers' having $/R_x/, /R_y/$ or $/R_z/>2.0$. It shows that if $/R_z/$ was <2.0 whilst both $/R_x/$ and $/R_y/$ were greater than 2.0 then when the values of d were between 2.6 and 2.8 g/dl, there was likely to have been a calibrator error only, but when d was < 2.6 g/dl or >2.8 g/dl both calibrator and zero setting of the analytical system were probably at fault.

In each trial the same sequence of exhaustive analysis is repeated for each parameter. Every participant receives a report giving assessments of his performance together with the grade A weighted means and standard deviations for the methods in which he reports (Fig. 6.6a). As an indication of national performance, the report includes a summary of the distribution, by method, of overall indices for each preparation together with the all-method values, noting the maximum and minimum values reported (Fig. 6.6b). Participants returning data for which $/R/>2.0$ are listed for long-term evaluation of their performance. It is also possible to compare methods using the trial data (Table 6.4). As inter-method comparability is excellent deterioration in the product is readily detected. For example a variant of ACD originally used at the East Anglian Blood Transfusion Centre (EABTC), was shown to alter the samples. As a result they responded differently to different test systems such that the apparent values for some parameters (MCV and PCV) varied between different methods (Fig. 6.7).

DHSS (LDAG) AND BCSH HEMATOLOGY QUALITY ASSESSMENT TRIAL 77-15 (NOVEMBER, '77) X = 771501, Y = 771502, Z = Y/X BLOOD COUNT

REPORT FOR LABORATORY 28

METHOD: SEMI-AUTOMATED

	SAMPLE X = 771501 YOUR SAMPLE WAS GRADE A				SAMPLE Y = 771502 YOUR SAMPLE WAS GRADE A			
	GRADE 'A' DATA		YOUR	INDEX	GRADE 'A' DATA		YOUR	INDEX
INVESTIGATION	MEAN	S.D.	RESULT	(/RX/)*	MEAN	S.D.	RESULT	(/RY/)*
HB (G/DL)	11.46	0.26	11.9	1.68	8.69	0.21	9.2	2.43
RBC (X10*12/LITRE)	5.184	0.294	5.410	0.77	3.888	0.250	4.000	0.45
PCV	0.334	0.009	0.329	0.57	0.255	0.009	0.254	0.14
MCV (FL)	64.66	3.74	60.8	1.03	65.21	3.61	63.5	0.47
MCH (PG)	22.12	1.15	22.0	0.10	22.43	1.44	23.0	0.40
MCHC (G/DL)	34.17	1.13	36.2	1.79	33.94	1.19	36.2	1.90
WBC (X10*9/LITRE)	24.44	1.57	26.1	1.05	23.08	1.37	24.5	1.04
	MEAN VARIANCE INDEX (/RO/)			1.00				0.98

METHOD: SEMI-AUTOMATED COMPUTED PCV

	SAMPLE X = 771501 YOUR SAMPLE WAS GRADE A				SAMPLE Y = 771502 YOUR SAMPLE WAS GRADE A			
	GRADE 'A' DATA		YOUR	INDEX	GRADE 'A' DATA		YOUR	INDEX
INVESTIGATION	MEAN	S.D.	RESULT	(/RX/)*	MEAN	S.D.	RESULT	(/RY/)*
HB (G/DL)	11.45	0.26	11.9	1.71	8.70	0.22	9.2	2.25
RBC (X10*12/LITRE)	5.331	0.125	5.410	0.63	4.016	0.079	4.000	0.20
PCV	0.344	0.010	0.372	2.70	0.263	0.008	0.279	1.96
MCV (FL)	65.23	1.88	67.8	1.37	65.31	2.23	68.9	1.61
MCH (PG)	21.54	0.88	22.0	0.52	21.73	0.80	23.0	1.59
MCHC (G/DL)	33.27	1.18	32.0	1.07	32.87	1.39	33.0	0.09
WRC (X10*9/LITRE)	24.82	1.29	26.1	0.99	23.50	1.12	24.5	0.90
	MEAN VARIANCE INDEX (/RO/)			1.28				1.23

NOTES:
ASSESSMENT OF VARIANCE INDEX:— <0.5 EXCELLENT; 0.5–1.0 GOOD; 1.0–2.0 SATISFACTORY BUT BORDERLINE; >2.0 CHECK CALIBRATION, CHECK INSTRUMENTATION.

1.0/RX/ OR /RY/ IS EQUIVALENT TO 1.0 SD.

Fig. 6.6a Trial report.

STANDARDIZATION FOR ROUTINE BLOOD COUNTING 109

TABLE 1

OVERALL INDEX (/RO/) METHOD	0.0	0.2	0.4	0.6	0.8	1.0	1.2	1.4	1.6	1.8	2.0	3.0	>3.0	TOTAL
				NUMBER OF LABORATORIES IN GROUP										

SAMPLE X

FULLY-AUTOMATED	2	18	36	47	45	27	21	10	4	8	6	0	0	224
FULLY-AUTOMATED-SPUN PCV	0	0	1	3	2	3	0	2	0	0	0	0	0	11
MANUAL	7	20	54	42	14	11	13	8	12	3	1	8	8	193
SEMI-AUTOMATED	3	13	26	39	18	10	9	10	4	1	5	5	5	143
SEMI-AUTOMATED COMPUTED PCV	1	5	12	11	8	8	3	1	3	5	2	1		60

SAMPLE Y

FULLY-AUTOMATED	3	19	37	57	31	27	18	16	6	3	6	3	0	226
FULLY-AUTOMATED-SPUN PCV	0	0	3	4	2	0	1	1	0	0	0	0		11
MANUAL	6	14	30	49	43	10	13	5	8	1	8	6		193
SEMI-AUTOMATED	4	16	30	26	26	8	16	4	1	3	5	5		144
SEMI-AUTOMATED COMPUTED PCV	1	8	14	8	10	5	3	0	1	2	6	2		60

TABLE 2

	SAMPLE 771501 GRADE 'A' WEIGHTED DATA		FOR VALID DATA VALUES		SAMPLE 771502 GRADE 'A' WEIGHTED DATA		FOR VALID DATA VALUES	
INVESTIGATION	MEAN	S.D.	MINIMUM	MAXIMUM	MEAN	S.D.	MINIMUM	MAXIMUM
HB (G/DL)	11.508	0.225	8.500	12.800	8.732	0.179	6.800	11.200
RBC (X10*12/LITRE)	5.257	0.193	3.210	6.300	3.994	0.168	2.190	5.460
PCV	0.339	0.010	0.032	0.390	0.260	0.009	0.190	0.377
MCV (FL)	64.807	2.335	55.000	89.000	65.088	2.441	21.000	88.500
MCH (PG)	21.920	0.854	0.000	0.000	21.925	0.974	0.000	0.000
MCHC (G/DL)	33.783	1.011	0.000	0.000	33.404	1.167	0.000	0.000
WBC (X10*9/LITRE)	24.733	1.425	2.400	31.300	23.393	1.312	2.100	32.000

THE OVERALL GRADE 'A' NATIONAL MEANS AND S.D'S (TABLE 2) ARE LISTED SO THAT PARTICIPANTS MAY ASSESS THEIR OWN DATA IN TERMS OF THE OVERALL PATTERN. THIS DOES NOT IMPLY THAT THESE NATIONAL OVERALL VALUES ARE THE 'CORRECT RESULTS'. IN THE SAME TABLE ARE THE MAXIMUM AND MINIMUM VALUES RETURNED FOR ALL TESTS EXCEPT MCH AND MCHC ON GRADE 'A', 'B', 'C', AND 'D' SAMPLES.

Fig. 6.6b Trial report, summary of distribution of overall indices for various preparations.

Table 6.3 Diagnosis of causes of 'poor performance'.

Participant	Sample (g/dl) x	y	Ratio z = y/x	Difference (g/dl) d = x − y	Deviation index /R_x/	/R_y/	/R_z/	Comment x y z
Weighted mean (m')	12.53	9.82	0.783	2.78				
Coulter S Plus								
A	12.4	10.0	0.806	2.4	0.92	1.64	4.01★	→ ← ←
B	12.7	10.1	0.780	2.6	1.26	2.55★	0.60	← ← =
C	12.2	9.4	0.770	2.8	2.38★	3.78★	2.15★	← → →
D	12.0	9.6	0.800	2.4	3.84★	1.97	2.91★	→ → ←
E	12.2	9.6	0.787	2.6	2.38★	1.97	0.66	→ → =
F	12.9	10.1	0.783	2.8	2.72★	2.55★	0.02	← ← =
G	12.2	9.6	0.787	2.6	2.38★	1.97	0.66	→ → =
Coulter S5								
H	12.5	10.0	0.800	2.5	0.19	1.64	2.91★	= ← ←
I	12.7	10.1	0.795	2.6	1.26	2.55★	2.10★	← ← ←
J	12.9	10.0	0.775	2.9	2.72★	1.64	1.35	← ← →
Coulter S junior								
K	13.0	10.2	0.785	2.8	3.45★	3.45★	0.27	← ← =
L	12.6	9.7	0.770	2.9	0.53	1.07	2.27★	= → →
Ortho ELT8								
M	13.2	10.2	0.773	3.0	4.91★	3.45★	1.77	← ← →

★ shows intra-laboratory inconsistency
= approximates to group mean
← higher than group mean
→ lower than group mean

Table 6.4 Current inter-method comparisons after exclusion of outliers.

	Method	Hb (g/dl) No	m	s	RBC (x 10^{12}/l) No	m	s	PCV No	m	s	MCV (fl) No	m	s	WBC (x 10^9/l) No	m	s
Sample 1	C	71	9.85	0.21	66	5.47	0.23	66	0.293	0.013	63	53.90	2.08	70	4.54	0.33
	F	173	9.89	0.13	168	5.52	0.10	169	0.293	0.010	172	52.93	1.90	173	4.87	0.38
	H	6	9.93	0.24	6	5.43	0.33	6	0.290	0.016	6	55.17	5.72	6	4.10	1.38
	M	18	9.86	0.19	6	5.17	0.44	19	0.291	0.007	8	55.94	5.23	15	4.52	0.49
	S	80	9.89	0.21	44	5.43	0.27	75	0.291	0.008	42	53.57	2.41	76	4.57	0.34
Sample 2	C	66	13.18	0.18	64	4.35	0.13	66	0.396	0.017	62	90.58	2.41	68	24.51	1.04
	F	169	13.07	0.15	167	4.36	0.07	168	0.403	0.008	169	92.10	1.73	168	24.51	1.15
	H	5	13.02	0.20	5	4.48	0.26	5	0.400	0.016	5	89.56	8.20	5	24.18	3.21
	M	18	13.02	0.22	6	4.27	0.24	18	0.409	0.008	8	95.15	5.94	14	22.86	1.91
	S	77	13.11	0.24	43	4.18	0.12	68	0.412	0.007	40	95.32	3.51	77	24.00	1.12

C Semi-automated (computed PCV) e.g. Coulter ZF_6 system
F Fully-automated, off-line mixing (computed PCV) e.g. Coulter S system
H Fully-automated, on-line mixing (spun PCV) e.g. Technicon Hemalog 8/90
M All fully manual techniques e.g. Visual counting
S Semi-automated (spun PCV) e.g. Coulter ZB_I with micro-haematocrit

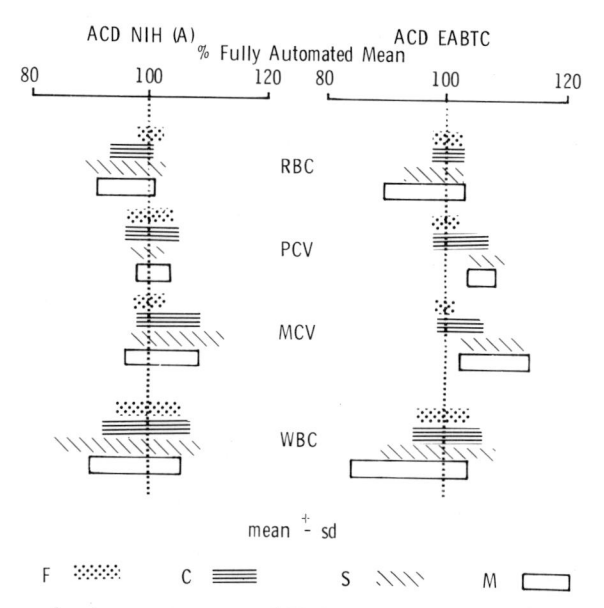

Fig. 6.7 Response of various test systems to ACD NIH-A and ACD EABTC when analyzing whole blood. F: Fully automated (computed PCV). C: Semi automated (computed PCV). S: Semi automated (spun PCV). M: Manual.

RECOGNITION OF POOR PERFORMANCE

Whilst statistical analysis of results in EQA trials provides a method for assessing reliability in performing a particular test, it is not necessarily the best method for judging poor performance in practice. This should also take account of the clinical relevance of measurement deviation and the extent of deviation of a measurement by an individual laboratory from the 'true' value as defined by definitive estimation and/or referee laboratories. The usefulness and limitations of these aspects will be considered below.

Statistical analysis

If it were accepted that poor performance was revealed by a result outside the range $m \pm 2SD$, then this would include 5 per cent of perfectly acceptable results in any trial. This 5 per cent is part of the Normal distribution and would persist however good the laboratories became. Therefore only when a laboratory is in the outer 5 per cent on several occasions would it be fair to regard this as 'poor performance'. When this occurs plotting data on a cumulative chart showing the overall deviation index /R/ (Fig. 6.8) may help in recognizing the origin of a fault. By looking at individual parameters it may be possible to identify particular errors, for example, low results on microcytic bloods due to incorrect threshold calibration. Similarly, on systems where the MCV is computed, a correct MCV but erroneous Hb and a red cell count suggests a constant dilution error.

When /R/>3.0 for at least one parameter in three consecutive trials the participant is contacted by the organizers of the EQA scheme on an informal basis

Examples of Laboratory Performance as assessed by overall Deviation Index (/R$_0$/)

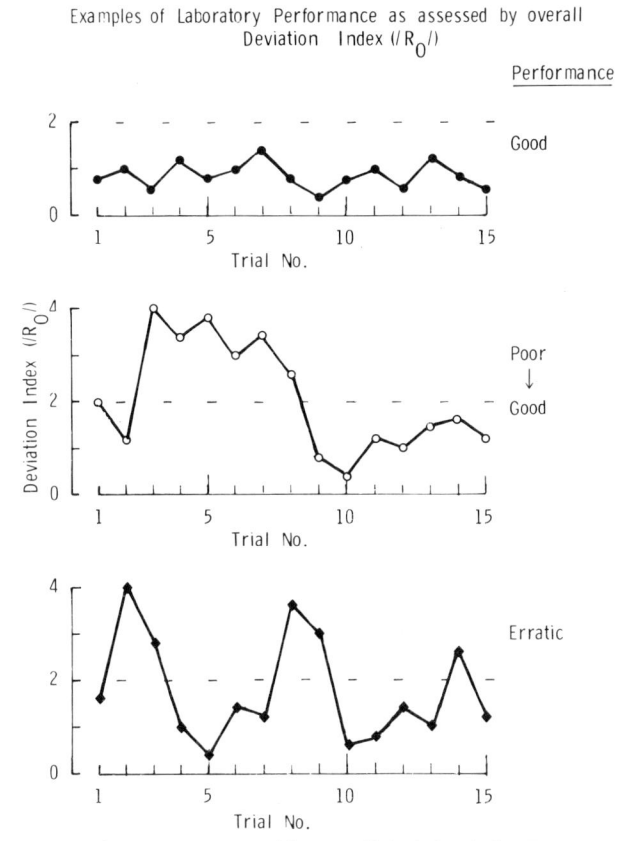

Fig. 6.8 Laboratory performance as assessed by overall deviation index /R$_0$/. (a) Consistently good performance (b) poor performance improving (c) erratic performance.

and invited to discuss the problem. Material is provided to help check instrument calibration and this usually improves performance. If the unsatisfactory performance continues the problem is then referred, by agreement between participant and organizer, to the National Advisory Panel which has been established jointly by the Royal College of Pathologists, the British Society for Haematology and the Institute of Medical Laboratory Sciences. It then becomes the responsibility of the Panel to try to solve the problem and improve the performance of the laboratory.

Clinical significance

The simple use of statistics can become unrealistic as performance in general improves. For example, in the UK scheme, precision has become so good that in the case of hemoglobin, a laboratory which differs from the mean by no more than 0.2 g/dl could be classified as a poor performer. It is therefore important to take account of the clinical relevance of an error and its potential effect on patient care. Although a 10 to 15 per cent error in hemoglobin concentration might not influence clinical decision, a similar difference in the prothrombin time may result in an inappropriate level of therapy. Thus, in anticoagulant control more rigid criteria must be applied than for the blood count. Defining acceptable performance in clinical terms must also take account of physiological variation and any other factors which, in practice, would be automatically discounted when analyzing the results of the laboratory tests. In practice, therefore, poor performance may best be defined as a result which could lead to inappropriate clinical action.

Target values
In hematology there are no definitive methods, apart from hemoglobinometry, by which we can establish values with certainty. It is a matter of debate whether it is more reliable to establish 'truth' on the basis of the statistical consensus described above, on the basis of results from a small number of selected laboratories of known reputation, or even on the results from one single 'reference' laboratory of unchallengeable reliability (if such exists). Taking account of the laborious procedure required for reference hemocytometry, there is much to be said for using the statistics from all participants to establish mean values, and for deviation based on clinical significance to assess poor performance. The great advantage of this approach is that it encourages a common level of standardization. A potential disadvantage of using the mean of results from a majority of participants to define the 'true' value is the fact that a result so obtained is not necessarily more accurate than that obtained by the other participants, as it is possible that the majority of results may be biased by a particular instrument type or calibration material if one such is used extensively throughout the country. This problem will be overcome only with the introduction of certified reference materials and recognition of the fact that many of the materials now used for calibration purposed should be regarded only as control materials.

CONCLUSION

For the laboratory to fulfill its role in patient care it must maintain a high level of proficiency. To achieve this requires an awareness of standardization and quality assurance. Because the ultimate concern relates to patients and not to specimens per se, laboratory proficiency should start with collection of the specimens from the patients and end only when the results generated in the laboratory have been presented to the physician in a way which can be easily comprehended and interpreted and with an assurance of their reliability, accuracy and clinical usefulness. Above all, it behoves the laboratory to apply internal quality control procedures at all times, for every test which is undertaken, and also to participate in external quality assessment schemes at national and regional levels.

National external quality assessment schemes have been established in many countries and are becoming recognized as an essential part of good laboratory practice. The good effect which this can have is illustrated in the measurement of hemoglobin by the laboratories in the UKEQA Scheme. When the scheme was started the CV for this estimate was 7 to 8 per cent but this has been progressively reduced to only 1.3 per cent (Fig. 6.9). Nevertheless, in each trial there are a few outliers whose results are seriously erroneous, thus highlighting

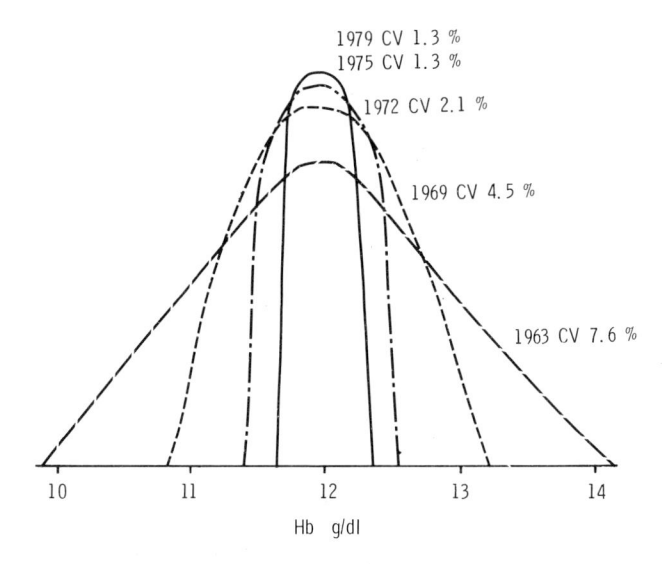

Fig. 6.9 Improvement in coefficient of variation on UKEQAS trial performance 1963–1979.

the need for constant vigilance if the high standard which has been achieved is to be maintained.

APPENDIX

METHODS FOR PREPARATION OF CONTROL MATERIAL

Human or equine blood is collected into ACD(NIH-A) or CPD and passed through a blood administration set to remove any clots. One unit (500 ml) of blood will provide, after preparative procedures, about 75 ml of lysate, 200 ml of resuspended fixed red cells or 500 ml of preserved blood.

1. Hemolysate
   1.1 Centrifuge blood at c 2000 g for 20 minutes and remove the plasma aseptically. This can be used subsequently for other quality control purposes.
   1.2 Add to each red cell deposit an equal volume of physiological saline (9 g/l w/v aqueous NaCl), mix well, transfer to a conventional centrifuge bottle and re-centrifuge; then discard the supernatant and the 'buffy coat'.
   1.3 Repeat saline wash three times to ensure complete removal of plasma, white cells and platelets.
   1.4 Add to the washed cells half their volume of toluene, cap and then shake vigorously on a mechanical shaker or vibrator for one hour: refrigerate overnight to allow the lipid/cell debris to form a semi-solid interface between toluene and lysate.
   1.5 On the following day centrifuge as before (1.1), remove toluene and into a clean bottle, syphon the lysate from under the lipid/cell debris using a

gentle water pump vacuum: re-centrifuge to extract more lysate and syphon off: finally centrifuge the combined lysate, and by vacuum suction remove residual lipid cell debris from the surface of the lysate.

1.6 Using gentle water pump suction, filter the centrifuged lysate through Whatman No. 42 filter paper in a Buchner funnel, changing the paper whenever the filtration slows down. It is important not to overload the funnel with lysate.

1.7 To each 70 ml of lysate add 30 ml glycerol and to each 500 ml of glycerol-lysate add one vial of penicillin-streptomycin, e.g. Crystamycin (Glaxo). Mix well; and then add 30 per cent v/v glycerol in 9 g/l NaCl containing antibiotic to the concentrated lysate to lower the hemoglobin concentration, as required. Store at 4°C until required for dispensing.

1.8 Pool the lysates into a mixing unit[4,6], mix well and dispense aseptically into sterile containers*; cap and seal with 'Viskrings'.[†]

1.9 To assign a value for hemoglobin content, use the reference method of spectrophotometric analysis of hemiglobincyanide checked against the ICSH international reference preparation or a secondary reference preparation derived from it.[7] Establish the CV by 10 replicate tests, sampling from several tubes taken at random from the batch. The CV should be less than ± 2 per cent. Check sterility in one of the tubes. Stored at 4°C, the product should maintain its assigned value for at least two years.

2. Fixed red cells[8]

Reagents:

0.15M iso-osmotic phosphate buffer (pH 7.4)
(A) — 23.4 g/l sodium dihydrogen phosphate ($Na_2HPO_4.2H_2O$)
(B) — 21.3 g/l anhydrous disodium hydrogen phosphate (Na_2HPO_4) or 53.7 g/l $Na_2HPO_4.12H_2O$ or 26.7 g/l $N_2HPO_4.2H_2O$ or 26.1 g/l K_2HPO_4
Both stock solutions keep well when refrigerated.
To 18 ml solution A add 82 ml solution B and mix well.

0.25 per cent glutaraldehyde fixative
To 1 l of phosphate buffer, add 5 ml 50 per cent glutaraldehyde solution (commercially available), mix by shaking and use at once.

12.5 per cent glycine solution
Dissolve 12.5 g glycine in distilled water and make to 100 ml. Store in refrigerator. This is a nearly saturated solution.

Antibiotic
Penicillin-streptomycin, e.g. Crystamycin (Glaxo)

2.1 Centrifuge blood at c 2000 g for 20 minutes and remove plasma aseptically for other uses.

2.2 Add equal volume of phosphate buffer to the red cells, mix and trans-

---

* γ-irradiated containers are available from most laboratory suppliers. Autoclaving and dry heat sterilization distorts many containers and caps.
† Viskrings — Viscose Development Co. Ltd., Croydon, Surrey, UK.

STANDARDIZATION FOR ROUTINE BLOOD COUNTING   117

fer to centrifuge bottle: re-centrifuge and discard supernatant and buffy coat.

2.3 Repeat wash and centrifugation twice.

2.4 Add to the washed red cells ten times their volume of glutaraldehyde fixative, mix by vigorous shaking to ensure complete resuspension and rotate slowly on a mechanical mixer for one hour. To test for complete fixation centrifuge 2 to 3 ml of the suspension, discard supernatant, add water to the deposit, mix and centrifuge, if hemolysis occurs, fixation is incomplete. Either more time is required or the stock glutaraldehyde requires replacement.

2.5 When fixation is complete, centrifuge the suspension at c 2000 g for 10 minutes and discard supernatant.

2.6 Add an equal volume of distilled water to the fixed cell deposit, resuspend and mix by stirring and shaking: again centrifuge at c 2000 g for 10 min and discard supernatant. Repeat twice.

2.7 Resuspend the fixed cells in the required volume of 12.5 per cent glycine (see 2.8) and mix well by vigorous shaking; place on a mechanical shaker for 24 hours to break up microclumps. The addition of a few 8 mm diameter glass beads speeds up this process.

2.8 Count levels above 2.5×10^{12} cells/l are difficult to resuspend. If a lower cell concentration is required add extra glycine solution. Add one vial of antibiotic for every 500 ml of suspension. Mix well. If necessary, store in refrigerator until required.

2.9 If the material has been stored, resuspend by vigorous hand shaking, followed by mechanical shaking until no clumps remain at the base of the bottle, transfer to mixing unit and mix for at least 20 minutes before dispensing into sterile containers, each of which contains two or three 3 mm glass beads to assist sample resuspension. Cap and seal with 'Viskrings.'

2.10 Establish the cell count value by 5 replicate hemocytometry estimations and/or 10 estimates on a standardized electronic cell counter.[9] Check dispensing by repeated counts on 5 or more randomly selected tubes. In each case the CV should be less than 3 per cent. Check sterility in one of the tubes.

2.11 For analysis, resuspend by vigorous hand shaking or vortex mixing and place on a mechanical mixer for at least 10 minutes before opening the tube. The unopened vials should be stable for several years.

Note: undiluted fixed cells are not suitable for use in fully automated systems

3. 'Pseudo-white' cells

As chicken and turkey red blood cells are nucleated, they are suitable for fixing to act as 'pseudo-white' cells in preserved whole bloods. For this purpose it is sufficient to collect 25 ml of blood into ACD (NIH-A) and process as for fixed red cells (see 2). This quantity of blood is sufficient for many trial preparations.

3.1 Reagent and procedure as for fixed red cells (sections 2.1 to 2.8).

3.2 Before use, resuspend by vigorous hand shaking followed by mechanical mixing until no clumps remain at the base of the container. Transfer the required volume of suspension to bulk diluent (3.3), mix well and dispense.

3.3 Although the 'pseudo-white' cell concentrate (c 2.5 × 10^{12}/l) is unsuitable for fully automated systems, no problems occur when it is diluted in preserved whole blood (4.2), added to hemolysate (see 1) for simultaneous control of Hb and WBC; or after diluting appropriately in 0.9 per cent saline.

3.4 Establish the cell count by five replicate hemocytometry estimations and/or 10 estimates by a standardized electronic cell counter.[9] Check the dispensing by repeated counts on five or more randomly selected tubes. The CV should be less than 5 per cent. Check sterility in one of the tubes.

3.5 For analysis, resuspend by the appropriate procedure (2.11 or 4.7). The shelf life of the unopened vials depends on the supporting diluent, i.e. blood, hemolysate or. saline.

4. Preserved blood[2]

Human blood is collected from one or more hepatitis Bs antigen negative donors of the same blood group in separate 500 ml donations. Equine blood may be collected in bags of up to 2 l capacity. Equine blood has been reported as hepatitis Bs free and we have no evidence of its presence in the donkeys and horses used in the UKEQA scheme.

4.1 Run the blood through blood administration sets directly into the mixing unit[4,6] and continue mixing for at least 20 minutes after the addition of the last unit of blood or other additives.

4.2 Red cell and white cell levels are adjusted as follows:
   a. To increase red cell count — sediment cells over exit vents of pack and run into mixer with minimum of plasma.
   b. To lower red cell count — add 0.9 per cent saline containing corresponding anticoagulant preservative, or add plasma of the same group.
   c. To raise white cell count — inject fixed avian cells (prepared as in 3 above) whilst blood is still running into mixer.
   d. To lower white cell count — pass blood through a leukocyte filter (Leuco-Pak Fenwal).

4.3 Add one vial of antibiotic for every 500 ml total volume whilst blood is running into mixer unit[4,6].

4.4 Dispense in sterile containers; cap and seal with 'Viskrings'. Refrigerate until required.

4.5 Check one tube for sterility and, if human blood, another for the absence of hepatitis Bs antigen.

4.6 Assign values for Hb as in 1.9, RBC as in 2.10, WBC as in 3.4, PCV by 10 replicate measurements using the system on which this material will be used (on ACD blood this may not necessarily be the same as the microhematocrit corrected for trapped plasma). The CV should not exceed 2 per cent. Check dispensing by repeated counts on five or more randomly selected tubes.

4.7 For analysis, the sample should be gently mixed on a roller mixer or by hand before opening. Unopened vials of human blood keep in good condition for about three weeks at 4°C, and those of equine blood for up to three months.

5. Fixed platelets[10]

Reagents:
0.15 per cent glutaraldehyde in Isoton II (Coulter)
Add 3 ml 50 per cent glutaraldehyde to 1 l of Isoton II, and mix well. This reagent should be prepared and used immediately.

0.15 per cent glutaraldehyde in glycerol/Isoton II
To each 600 ml glycerol, add 400 ml Isoton II and 3 ml 50 per cent glutaraldehyde, and mix well. This reagent should also be used without delay.

Antibiotic
Penicillin-streptomycin, e.g. Crystamycin (Glaxo)

5.1 Centrifuge well mixed fresh blood at 200 *g* for 10 minutes and remove the platelet rich plasma.

5.2 Dispense 100 ml volumes of glutaraldehyde-Isoton II solution into a series of clean dry 150 ml screw-capped glass bottles and to each add 15 ml platelet rich plasma. Mix and cap. Roller mix for 20 minutes. (As the final platelet concentration in the plasma-glutaraldehyde-Isoton II mixture should not exceed about $250 \times 10^9/l$, less platelet-rich plasma must be used if it has a very high platelet content: larger volumes of fixative and plasma should not be mixed as this induces clumping.

5.3 Pool the suspensions in the flask of the mixing unit[4,6] which has previously been cooled and rotate at 4°C for 24 hours.

5.4 Pass the suspension through a 20 μm high capacity transfusion filter (Fenwal) to remove fibrin strands and any other debris.

5.5 Dispense 50 ml volumes of glutaraldehyde-glycerol-Isoton II solution into another set of 150 ml screw-capped bottles; carefully layer onto this solution 50 ml of filtered fixed platelet suspension and cap.

5.6 Stand at 4°C for four days to allow the fixed platelets to drift through the glycerol based mixture so that the initially yellowish supernatant becomes clear and the lower layer milky.

5.7 With gentle suction remove the supernatant and 2 to 3 ml of the lower layer.

5.8 Resuspend platelets by shaking and roller mix for 20 minutes before pooling in mixing unit[4,6] and after adding antibiotic (one vial to every 500 ml platelet suspension) dispense into sterile irradiated containers; seal with 'Viskrings'. Adjustment to platelet concentration is made by

removing more of the lower layer at 5.7 or by adding more of the glycerol-based mixture.
5.9 Check sterility.
5.10 Assign values by five hemocytometer counts using the reference method.[9] An electronic counter may be used to check dispensing by repeated counts on a number of randomly selected tubes (at least five). The CV in both cases should not exceed 3 per cent.

REFERENCES

1. Lewis S M, Burgess B J 1969 Quality control in haematology: report of interlaboratory trials in Britain. British Medical Journal iv: 253–256
2. Lewis S M 1975 Standards and reference preparations. In: Lewis S M, Coster J F (eds) Quality control in haematology. Academic Press, New York, p 79–95
3. Morgan L O, Jones W G, Fisher J, Cavill I 1900 A whole blood control for the Coulter Model S. Journal of Clinical Pathology 31: 50–53
4. Ward P G, Chappell D A, Fox J G C, Allen B V 1975 Mixing and bottling unit for preparing biological fluids used in quality control. Laboratory Practice 24: 577–583
5. Ward P G, Lewis S M 1975 Interlaboratory trials — a national proficiency assessment scheme for Britain. In: Lewis S M, Coster J F (eds) Quality control in haematology. Academic Press, New York, p 37–51
6. Chappell D A, Ward P G 1978 Safe and sterile mixer for biological fluids. Laboratory Equipment Digest 16: 75–77
7. International Committee for Standardization in Haematology 1978 Recommendations for reference method for haemoglobinometry in human blood (ICSH Standard EP 6/2: 1977) and specifications for international haemiglobincyanide reference preparation (ICSH Standard EP 6/3: 1977) Journal of Clinical Pathology 31: 139–143.
8. Archer R K, Lewis S M, Burgess B J 1970 Red cell suspensions as a reference in blood counting. In: Astaldi G, Sirtoric, Vanzetti G (eds) Standardization in haematology. Franco Angeli Editore, Milan, p 175–180
9. Van Assendelft O W, England J M 1981 Advances in hematological methods: the blood count. CRC Press, Boca Raton Florida.
10. Lewis S M, Wardle J, Cousing S, Skelly J 1979 Platelet counting — development of a reference method and a reference preparation. Clinical and Laboratory Haematology 1: 227–237

7
Intralaboratory Quality Control Using Patients' Data
B. S. Bull   R. A. Korpman

Whole blood is an extraordinarily complex suspension. Many of its components are highly unstable. As a consequence, the calibration and control of automated whole blood analyzers pose a problem that has yet to be resolved in a completely satisfactory manner. The approach of the purist is to recalibrate the machine several times daily with fresh whole blood samples which have been exhaustively analyzed by reference or by definitive methods. As might be anticipated, this approach is extremely time consuming. Furthermore, the performance of reference methods for the purpose of primary whole blood standardization is likely to be beyond the capability of just those laboratories where improvements are most needed.

Most laboratories are content, therefore, to rely upon purchased control materials that have been analyzed by the manufacturer. The analyzer is checked once or twice each 24 hours to be certain that the values obtained fall within the acceptable limits of the control material. This approach falls short of the ideal for several reasons. First, there may be problems in the control material itself. It may have been inadequately analyzed by the manufacturer, the values may have changed during shipment or storage because of exposure to temperature extremes, it may have a far shorter period of stability than the dating period implies or it may resuspend only by the application of such force that this is unlikely ever to be completed in the laboratory. Second, because of the expense involved, these materials are typically used far too infrequently. Many hours may elapse between quality control runs and many patient specimens are thus at risk of being incorrectly analyzed by a machine that has suffered an abrupt calibration loss. Finally, the majority of these preparations are designed for control, not for calibration, though this distinction is honored more in the breach than in the observance.

While it is seldom actually implemented, a combination of reference methods with purchased control material, comes closer to the ideal. In such a system each new lot of manufactured control material received in the laboratory would be assayed on an analyzer that has just been calibrated by the use of reference methods. The values would thus be assigned to the preparation at the point of use and all that would now be required of the control material is stability throughout the claimed dating period. This method of quality control would still require that the laboratory be able to skilfully carry out the whole blood reference methods, but the process would need to be done at intervals of weeks rather than days. There is a method of quality control which requires the performance reference methods at intervals of months or years rather than weeks and relies in the intervening periods not upon the stability of a partially stabilized whole blood suspension, but upon the stability of the mean erythrocyte indices of a patient population.

STABILITY, THE ESSENTIAL REQUIREMENT FOR HAEMATOLOGICAL QUALITY CONTROL

Stability is an absolute requirement for quality control. An analytical instrument must be stable for long enough to permit the analysis of a reasonable number of specimens between each calibration run. The calibration/control standards must be stable or they will be ineffective in translating definitive or reference methodology into unbiased machine calibration and control. So central is the issue of stability that it may be taken as the starting point for this discussion of quality control.

Instability of one sort or another underlies most of our present problems with quality control in· hematology. In clinical chemistry many of the analytes are either elements or well-defined chemical compounds which can be prepared in dry form and which, in that form, are stable indefinitely. This situation approaches the ideal. The analyte itself is stable and can be preserved almost indefinitely in a form identical with, or readily referable to, the form in which it is to be analyzed. In hematology the situation is much more bleak. There is only a single stable reference material — cyanmethemoglobin. This stable reference cannot be conveniently prepared in concentrations approaching those in which hemoglobin is present in whole blood. It can be easily prepared only in the far more dilute concentrations characteristic of a blood specimen already diluted for spectrophotometry. Thus, while the reference material serves to adequately control hemoglobin analyzer calibration, it does not, in the usual case, provide much help towards increasing the accuracy and the reproducibility of all of the preliminary steps that prepare a whole blood specimen for the spectrophotometric analysis.

As already noted hematology can boast of only a single stable reference material — cyanmethemoglobin. This paucity of stable reference material is the reason that such frequent recourse must be had to reference methods rather than to reference material. If fresh blood is analyzed by reference methodology, the resulting blood sample becomes a reference material, but its useful life is measured in hours because it is so unstable. If the same reference methods are applied to stabilized whole blood suspensions, the resultant material hardly qualifies as reference largely because the dating period, while longer than that of fresh whole blood, is still awkwardly short. A dating period of four to six weeks is barely long enough to permit the material to be shipped one way to the user and still have some time left within the dating period to permit the material to serve its intended purpose in the laboratory. Ideally, a reference material would be shipped to several reference laboratories and there it would be analyzed repetitively and exhaustively. Any discrepancies between reference laboratories would be resolved and then the material would be shipped to intermediates around the world who would transfer the accuracy of the primary reference material to stable secondary standards. These stable secondary standards would then be made available to each individual laboratory for use in quality control. Such a process would require that the reference material be stable for at least a year. Five- or ten-year stability would make the whole process even more feasible.

Surprisingly, the requisite stability of 12 months or more can be made available — not in the familiar form of liquid in a bottle, but in an unfamiliar though no less useful form. The red cell indices of hospitalized patients are stable over weeks, months and years.[1] That the indices should be so stable is not, upon reflection, surprising. The red cell indices are very tightly controlled physiologically, apparently because the red cell functions optimally only within a very narrow range of size and hemoglobin content. Nature, with characteristic parsimony, varies the number of red cells present to meet differing metabolic needs, but she does not trifle with the more fundamental properties of size and hemoglobin concentration.

Red cell indices in normal individuals vary with a coefficient of variation of about 4 per cent. In the patient population of a typical, acute care, general hospital the variation is only slightly greater, in the order of 6 per cent. The average of repeated estimates of a mean will have a coefficient of variation (CV) which is reduced in inverse proportion to the square root of the number of items averaged. With 100 patient samples included for each mean the CV of 6 per cent becomes a CV of 0.6 per cent for variation in the means. Thus it is that if the red cell indices of individual patients are averaged by finding the mean indices of a population of 100 or more patients, the stability of that mean, or to express it more conventionally the CV of that mean, will be well under 1 per cent. This, then, is a stable reference point in the hematology laboratory.

The RBC indices of a population represent numerical values that can be readily calculated and which will vary no more than 0.5 per cent from day to day, month to month and year to year, providing the population does not change its characteristics.

STABILITY OF THE RED CELL INDICES VERSUS STABILITY OF THE HEMOGLOBIN, HEMATOCRIT AND RED CELL COUNT

The knowledge that the red cell indices of a population are highly stable does not, in itself, help very much in hematological quality control. It is the primary measurements which usually interest the physician and which typically are the precipitating cause for the analysis of the blood sample. The hemoglobin, packed cell volume and red cell count are the results of interest. These are the test methods for which quality control is desired. Compared to the primary measurements the red cell indices are less useful for the diagnosis of disease and the monitoring of therapy for precisely the reasons that they are useful for quality control — because they are so stable. They remain unchanged during most nonhematological illnesses. They even remain stable in many patients suffering from hematological problems (macrocytic and microcytic anemias being the most obvious exceptions). The reason why the six red cell related parameters — Hb, RBC, PCV, MCV, MCH, and MCHC — can be divided so unequivocally into two groups on the issue of stability is worth exploring further. The reasons underlying this dichotomy are fundamental to understanding the means by which patients' data can be used for quality control.

The first and most obvious difference between the indices and the primary measurements is that the former are all ratios whereas the latter are not. Provided the two primary determinations on which an index is based are both measured on aliquots from the same primary dilution, the accuracy of that index will be unaffected even by gross errors in dilution. Inadequate mixing of a blood specimen prior to analysis has no effect on the measurement of the red cell indices of that sample. The same immunity from dilutional or mixing error does not extend to the primary measurements upon which the indices are based.

There is a second reason for the stability of the indices when compared to the primary measurements. Physiological control mechanisms first modify red cell number in the regulation of red cell mass to meet varying tissue oxygen needs. Only when physiological response mechanisms are overwhelmed does the bone marrow start to modify red cell size and hemoglobin content. The humoral effects that bring about differences in the mean hemoglobin levels between males and females fall well within the physiological response of normal bone marrow. As a consequence, the response of the marrow is limited to adjustment of cell number. The same can be said of the majority of illnesses.

To reiterate, the indices reflect red cell size and hemoglobin content. Both of these parameters are controlled with exquisite precision by bone marrow physiological mechanisms. Furthermore, the indices are ratios and thus are independent of many of the procedural errors that degrade the primary measurements. Unfortunately, it is the primary measurements which are most useful clinically and also most in need of quality control. How can the stability of the indices be used to decrease the variability and increase the accuracy of, for example, the red cell count?

STABILITY TRANSLATED INTO UTILITY

The fact that each index is a ratio is a decided advantage if stability is desired. It is a disadvantage when data from the indices is to be used for quality control of the primary measurements. Consider for a moment what would happen to the MCV or MCH of each blood sample analyzed on a machine that was underdiluting by 50 per cent. The indices would be unaffected (assuming, of course, that the analyzer was linear over the concentration range involved). The hemoglobin, packed cell volume and red cell count, on the other hand, would be vastly overestimated. In fact, massive variability can occur in the primary determinations without affecting either the individual sample indices or the mean indices of a patient population, provided that all of the primary determinations vary synchronously with each other. If the error in all three primary measurements is quantitatively similar and in the same direction, then no error will be introduced into the indices. For this reason, correct indices are no guarantee of correct calibration unless it is known that one of the primary measurements — Hb, PCV or RBC — is also correct. In theory, any one of the three is equally serviceable for this purpose. In practice, the hemoglobin determination is the one most frequently used.

In order to exercise quality control over the six red cell related measurements, some way must be found to directly validate at least three of those measurements. If the quality control scheme is of the traditional type, then a stable, calibrating substance must be employed that permits validation of the Hb, the RBC and the PCV. A quality control program based on patients' data provides alternatives for two of the three measurements to be directly validated. Hb is common to both approaches, but any two of the three indices — MCV, MCH or MCHC — can be used instead of the RBC and PCV. The inherent stability of the mean red cell indices in the population provides the quality control 'substances', to substitute for a stabilized blood sample of constant RBC and PCV. The only bottled quality control material that is now required is cynamethemoglobin — a material that is stable, inexpensive and readily available. While only two of the red cell indices are required (the third can always be calculated given any two), it is convenient to plot all three. These plots facilitate pattern recognition and readily identify those occasions when results are incorrect not because the analyzer has drifted, but because of faulty computation of a particular index.

It is not necessary to pick the hemoglobin assay as the one primary determination to be standardized by comparison with a known true reference. Hemoglobin is usually chosen because of the ready availability of a stable standard. Once the decision is made as to which primary measurement is to be used and the bias (if any) of this measurement determined, the bias in the indices is measured simply by comparing the figures obtained on the last batch or batches of patient mean indices to the known true mean indices of the whole patient population. This operation presupposes that the mean indices have been estimated correctly from some randomly selected, conveniently small number of blood samples, and that the true mean indices of the entire population have been accurately determined. How to perform each of these two tasks is discussed in the next two sections.

UNBIASED ESTIMATES OF MEAN RED CELL INDICES FROM SMALL RANDOM SAMPLES

Achieving an unbiased estimate of the red cell indices of a population is rendered difficult by the boundary conditions noted in the heading for this section. The sample must be small and randomness is required to ensure that the estimate is unbiased. Unlike the 'true' red cell indices, the term 'observed indices' used in this section refers to what the indices of the patient population would appear to be if the individual patient indices had been measured on the analyzer under study. The two sets of indices (the observed and the true or target indices) will be identical only if the analyzer being used is calibrated correctly.

For quality control purposes the smaller the number of patient samples required for each estimate the better. Why is this so? The smaller the batch size, the more frequently the estimates of the mean indices are available, the greater the potential for 'tight' quality control. An analyzer frequently loses calibration via a slow drift. If the batch size is small, the calibration can be corrected at shorter intervals and the average machine bias will be lessened. If the analyzer loses correct calibration by an abrupt shift in one or more of the analytical channels, then the time interval before that calibration loss can be identified and corrected is directly proportional to the number of samples which must be analyzed before the next estimate of the state of calibration can be made.

Ideally, the batch size should be a single sample. Averages require at least two samples. How many more than two will be required depends in very large measure on the type of statistical treatment accorded the data. For the red cell indices an arithmetical average of the data from 100 or more patients will provide mean values that are stable enough to be highly useful for quality control. But, 100 patients is an inconveniently large sample. In many laboratories it would limit quality control estimates to no more than one per day. If the analyzer were then found to be in error, an entire day's run would have been incorrectly analyzed.

A batch size of far less than 100 patients can be successfully employed with statistical averaging techniques that are more powerful than the simple arithmetic mean. All of the algorithms employed for this purpose decrease the variance of the estimated means. They, in effect, make a small batch of data behave statistically like a much larger data batch. Using these techniques, it is possible to analyze the data from 15 to 20 patients and estimate the means of the red cell indices as reproducibly and accurately as if 80 to 100 patients were analyzed by a simple arithmetic averaging procedure.

Of the several algorithms available,[2] the one that has been most extensively used for this purpose is:[3]

$$\overline{X}_{B,i} = \overline{X}_{B,i-1} + \text{sgn}\left(\sum_{j=1}^{N}\text{sgn}(X_{ji} - \overline{X}_{B,i-1})\sqrt{|X_{ji} - \overline{X}_{B,i-1}|}\right) \times \frac{\left(\sum_{j=1}^{N}\text{sgn}(X_{ji} - \overline{X}_{B,i-1})\sqrt{|X_{ji} - \overline{X}_{B,i-1}|}\right)^2}{N}$$

This algorithm contributes to a reduction in variability through two mechanisms. First, it markedly reduces the contribution of outliers — values far removed from the mean. Second, it incorporates information from the preceeding means into the estimate of the present mean and thus, like a moving average, dampens any large shifts from one mean to the next. On inspection of the algorithm, the basis for these two effects can be seen. Each incoming data item is compared to the mean of all items of the same type in the preceeding batch. The square root of the absolute value of this difference is then taken. This markedly diminishes the extent to which an abnormal sample can influence the mean of the 19 other samples in the batch. Furthermore, the magnitude of the difference of each item is determined by comparison with the mean of the preceeding batch. In this fashion, information from the preceeding batch (and all of the batches before it) is included in the process.

The algorithm has another characteristic which increases its usefulness for quality control purposes. If it is compared to a simple arithmetic mean under circumstances where an abrupt shift in machine calibration takes place between one data batch and another, the algorithm will reflect less of a shift than the arithmetic mean. The amount that it underestimates the true extent of the shift increases with increasing variance within the second batch of data. In effect, the algorithm adopts a 'wait and see' attitude towards an abrupt data shift, particularly when the data batch which first indicates the shift has a large standard deviation due to the presence of many outliers. If, on the other hand, the first data batch reflecting an abrupt shift has a very tight data distribution with a small standard deviation, the algorithm will quantitatively reflect virtually all of the shift in the new mean calculated from that data batch. The more reliable the data, the more responsive the algorithm becomes.

The application of an averaging algorithm makes it possible to estimate the means of the red cell indices on sample sizes of 15 to 20 while staying within useful limits of variability. What about the requirement that the small sample be randomly selected? This requirement is absolute. Even sophisticated averaging techniques cannot compensate for non-randomness in the raw data. If all 20 patients included in a sample are on cancer chemotherapy or are neonates, then all of the patients are likely to have increased MCVs and MCHs. An average of these same 20 patients will show a similar increase. The increase on Coulter® analyzers is indistinguishable from a calibration loss due to protein buildup in the RBC aperture tubes. The confusion does not pose an insurmountable problem, but it does require time and attention whenever it occurs. For this reason it is highly desirable to ensure that samples are randomized prior to analysis at least to the extent that no more than one third of the samples in any one batch come from a cancer chemotherapy ward, a neonatal unit or an iron deficiency anemia clinic. Fortunately, once this problem has been solved it usually stays solved. If the appropriate randomization procedures have been incorporated into the normal specimen handling routines of a particular laboratory, adequate randomization is usually assured for months to years.

DETERMINING THE 'TRUE' (TARGET) RED CELL INDICES OF A POPULATION

Intralaboratory quality control based on patients' samples requires comparison of the means of small, random subsets to the real means of that same patient population. This operation presupposes that the real mean values have been measured. This process, though time consuming, would appear to be simple to execute. As will shortly become apparent, it is a more complex process than it appears to be. It may, in fact, lie beyond the capacity of many laboratories if it is to be performed in an uncompromising manner.

Ideally, the process of determining the true red cell indices of a patient population begins with a meticulous calibration of the whole blood analyzer (Ch. 2). Using reference methods,[4] several fresh whole blood samples are analyzed and these in turn are used as calibrators to set the various analytical channels on the whole blood analyzer. The most common point of failure in this process comes in the performance of the red cell count. Failure to perform an accurate red cell count will render impossible an accurate assessment of the mean red cell indices of the population. Once calibrated, the state of calibration is checked at least daily by including further samples that have been measured by the reference methods. The analyzer is, by this means, kept correctly calibrated until more than 500 patient samples have been analyzed by the automated blood counter. The red cell indices from these samples are then averaged. An arithmetic mean is entirely adequate for this step because the large number of samples ensures randomness. The resultant mean MCV, MCH and MCHC are, if the process has been correctly performed, the 'true' mean indices for that patient population. Their stability can be relied upon for months to years.

As an alternative, the red cell indices can be assumed to be identical with those observed in other similar populations. This approach is not as perilous as it might appear to be at first glance. Those patient populations in acute general care hospitals which we have been studying have been consistently similar with respect to their red cell indices. Furthermore, a slight overestimate or underestimate of the true red cell indices will have no significant effect on patient management within a particular hospital. Only when the data obtained on a particular patient at one hospital is used to modify the care of that patient at another hospital would any effect be detectable. Under these circumstances there are other factors operating which will overwhelm any effects from minor inaccuracies in the assumed red cell indices. Some laboratories routinely apply a trapped plasma correction to the blood samples which they analyze. Other laboratories do not. In those laboratories where trapped plasma corrections are used, the extent of the correction varies from approximately 1 per cent to 3 per cent. In other laboratories a trapped plasma correction is applied unwittingly. This occurs because a control material is being used (incorrectly) as a calibrator and the manufacturer of that material has incorporated a trapped plasma correction into the values assigned to the control material. Laboratories which rely for calibration upon such materials are, as a consequence, forced to accept whatever that particular manufacturer regards as appropriate in the way of a correction factor. As a result of these variations in trapped plasma correction factors, large uncertainties are introduced into estimates of the mean red cell indices by different laboratories. These variations effectively swamp any minor differences in patient population means — if such differences do indeed exist. Typical values for the three indices and acceptable ranges which will cover most trapped plasma corrections are illustrated in Table 7.1.

A compromise approach which is easy to implement and which effectively protects against the possibility that the population under study has unique and markedly different indices from those analyzed to date can be implemented

Table 7.1 Typical population mean values and acceptable ranges for the three red cell indices

Index	Typical value	Acceptable range
MCV	88.5	87 90
MCH	29.5	29 30.5
MCHC	33.5	33 34

in the following fashion. The analyzer in question should be calibrated using at least two separate lots of stabilized whole blood from one manufacturer or one lot from each of two manufacturers. This procedure should be repeated at least daily throughout the study period. After the first several hundred patient samples have been analyzed the mean indices should be determined by arithmetic averaging and compared with the values given in Table 7.1. If they correspond to one of the sets of data and if the trapped plasma correction that this implies is satisfactory, then those mean indices are the 'true' mean indices for that patient population. A different trapped plasma correction (or zero correction if desired) can be easily superimposed on the mean indices at this time. Only in the very rare instance that the mean indices fail to fall within the ranges given will it be necessary to go through the lengthy process of primary whole blood standardization. Before this process is undertaken, it would be prudent to look first for arithmetical errors or unstable instrumentation.

The prerequisites for a quality control scheme based on patients' data are at hand. The 'true' (target) mean indices of the patient population have been ascertained. Randomization of the incoming specimens has been assured by adjustments to the standard operating procedures of the venipuncturists. The appropriate algorithm has been selected. The quality control procedure is ready for implementation — but is it to be off line or on line?

OFF LINE IMPLEMENTATION OF QUALITY CONTROL BASED ON PATIENTS' DATA

This approach involves the least initial expense. An already programmed calculator can be purchased[5] or the user may elect to purchase a programmable calculator and to program the algorithm himself.[6] In daily operation, the indices of each patient sample are then entered manually on the calculator keyboard. This method can provide effective quality control for smaller laboratories processing relatively few (<100) blood counts each day. It does, however, have several inherent deficiencies. These stem from the time consuming nature of the manual data entry step and from the errors that are inevitably introduced by the transcription process.

The amount of technologist time required is usually about three minutes per batch of 20 patients. A simple cost analysis calculation will disclose the breakeven point for the particular workload handled by a particular laboratory. It is much more difficult to calculate the cost of the errors introduced by the data transcription process. Errors of data entry now become the most frequent cause of an apparent loss of machine calibration. Review of, and if necessary recalculation of, all 20 samples in the questionable data batch now becomes the most appropriate initial response to an apparent quality control problem. This process inevitably delays the recognition and complicates the correction of analyzer calibration changes.

If the data entry is completely manual, it is possible simply not to enter data from neonatal intensive care units or from physicians known to treat patients with hematological problems. This will partially compensate for the problems introduced by data transcription errors. Unsuspected clustering, in one data batch, of patient samples with abnormal indices now becomes an exceedingly unlikely cause of apparent loss of machine calibration. Either the analyzer has, in fact, lost calibration or erroneous data entry is the culprit.

ON LINE IMPLEMENTATION OF QUALITY CONTROL BASED ON PATIENTS' DATA

Even if the data on patient red cell indices is transferred automatically from the analyzer to the computational module, there are two points at which the process may take place. The most satisfactory point is after the data has been validated and is ready for inclusion into the patient record. It is less satisfactory to transfer all data as soon as available and rely on the operator to cancel data that arises from wash cycles, short samples, etc. This less than ideal approach (as is often the case) is cheaper. The required equipment consists of an interface and an appropriately matched programmable calculator. The calculator, for reasons already mentioned, must make it possible to eliminate from consideration the immediately upcoming result. It is also a convenience to be able to eliminate data from the most recent patient sample that has been accepted. The unsuitability of a particular analysis is often not appreciated until after the analysis is complete and the data has already been released to the calculator.

Quality control based on patients' data is optimally implemented on line through a processor that permits the data to be reviewed and validated prior to release. Ideally, acceptable data should be released simultaneously to the patient record and to the quality control computation. Such implementation requires either that the analyzer has its own data handler or that similar facilities be available on a laboratory computer. All laboratory computers are powerful enough to handle the necessary statistical manipulation and it seems likely that in the very near future all hematology analyzers will be also.

INITIATING AND RUNNING THE QUALITY CONTROL PROGRAM

The concepts and procedures outlined in this chapter lend themselves to presentation in the form of a flow chart. The chart (Fig.7.1) indicates the sequence followed in the implementation of this approach to quality control. The steps indicated along the margins of the flow chart are discussed in detail below.

Step I: enter the target means
The target means should be entered into the appropriate registers of the computational module. The target means are the values for MCV, MCH and MCHC which have been previously determined to be the true red cell indices of the patient population under analysis. These values will be compared with the observed means after each batch of n (typically 20) patients. Any difference,

assuming that it passes the screens imposed by Steps IV through VI, quantitatively reflects the bias present in a particular analytical module.

The algorithmn compares each patient index, such as the MCV, with the mean index of the preceeding patient batch. For this reason it is necessary, when initiating the calculations, to assume a value for preceding batch simply as a starting point. While any reasonable figure for each of the three indices will serve, the closer the starting figure is to the true mean of the patient population, the sooner the calculated means will actually reflect the patient data. For this reason, it is convenient to insert the target means into the appropriate computational module as starting values. Once patient data becomes available it will, of course, replace these assumed values and the observed indices will be the red cell indices of the patient samples being processed.

Step II: enter patient data; calculate the observed means
While the actual calculation of the observed mean values is performed by the computational module, the data entry step may require more or less attention depending upon the manner in which the quality control program has been implemented. Each data item consists of the red cell indices as calculated by the analyzer on each patient sample. If data input is manual, the three indices are first checked for reasonableness and then keyed into the computational module. If patient values from certain services and/or certain physicians are to be excluded from the computation, such values are eliminated at this point. This is the only form of data manipulation that should be employed. No other screens or thresholds should be applied and if some patients from certain services or wards are excluded, then all patients from that location should be excluded whether or not their indices appear to fall within normal limits.

With manual data entry programs all decisions to exclude certain data elements can be made prior to the data entry step. If the data is transfered automatically via an interface, then other potential ways of contaminating the data base still exist. With automatic data transfer the indices from incorrectly analyzed samples can get into the computation, as can spurious values from wash cycles, priming cycles, etc. Provision must be made in the programming for the elimination of these incorrect entries. This may appear to be a simple task; it is not. The spurious values must either be retrieved or their effects on the computation cancelled and the specimen counter decremented by one. If this is not done, then a single incorrect data entry will typically require the re-entry and recalculation of some 60 two-or-three-digit items. If another error is made on the second attempt, the process can go on for many minutes. This process is highly frustrating and quickly dampens enthusiasm for this approach to quality control. The ideal arrangement is the simultaneous release of validated patient data to the patient's medical record and to the computational module. All of the problems discussed above disappear and the computational process operates only on data of the highest possible quality.

Step III: compare observed means with target means
At this point the indices from each of n consecutive patient samples have been

132   QUALITY CONTROL

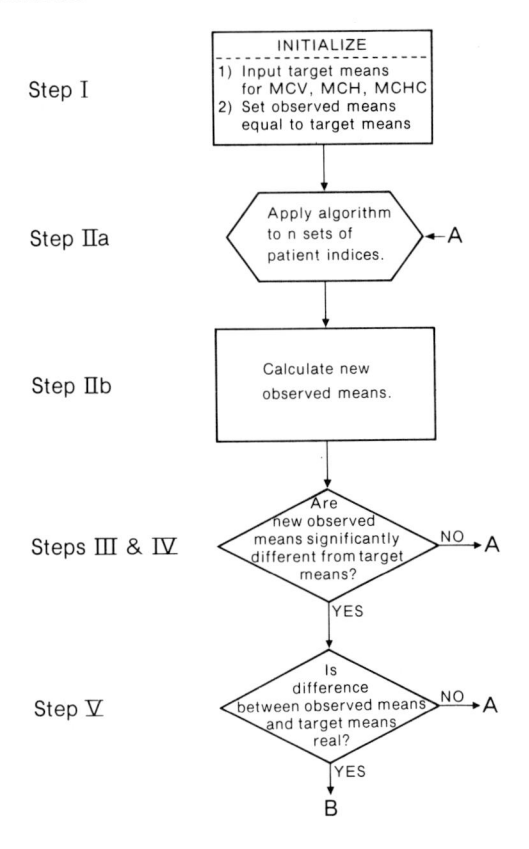

```
Step I            ┌─────────────────────────┐
                  │        INITIALIZE       │
                  │ 1) Input target means   │
                  │    for MCV, MCH, MCHC   │
                  │ 2) Set observed means   │
                  │    equal to target means│
                  └─────────────────────────┘
                              │
                              ▼
Step IIa            ╱ Apply algorithm ╲
                   ╱  to n sets of    ╲ ◄── A
                   ╲  patient indices. ╱
                    ╲                ╱
                              │
                              ▼
                  ┌─────────────────────────┐
Step IIb          │   Calculate new         │
                  │   observed means.       │
                  └─────────────────────────┘
                              │
                              ▼
                         ╱ Are     ╲
                        ╱ new observed╲
Steps III & IV         ╱ means significantly╲  NO
                       ╲ different from target╱ ──► A
                        ╲  means?  ╱
                         ╲        ╱
                           │ YES
                           ▼
                         ╱   Is    ╲
                        ╱ difference╲
Step V                 ╱ between observed means╲  NO
                       ╲  and target means    ╱ ──► A
                        ╲    real?  ╱
                         ╲        ╱
                           │ YES
                           ▼
                           B
```

Fig. 7.1 Flowchart for on-line implementation of quality control based on patients' data.

entered and the new mean indices have been calculated. These updated, observed means are now compared with the target means. If no difference exists, no further action is called for other than plotting the data and indicating that the data has been evaluated for quality control purposes. A convenient way of handling the data is illustrated in Figure 7.2. As illustrated, the graph allows 20 batches, each of 20 patients, to be plotted for a total of 400 patients. As the results from each batch of data are entered onto the quality control chart it is joined with the equivalent preceding result by a straight line. The upper and lower limits represent a deviation from the expected means of 3 per cent. Interpretation of the graphical patterns formed by the plots of the mean indices is significantly enhanced if quantitatively similar deviations in each of the indices are reflected by similar movements of the plot. For this reason the MCV result should be divided by three prior to plotting. This step makes it easier to average visually the last two or the last three data points to confirm that any change judged sufficiently large to require recalibration has persisted over more than a single batch of patient data. The technologist responsible for evaluating and plotting the data initials and dates each entry as it is made. This simple technique ensures that the quality control data is reviewed in a timely fashion and that the reviewer is identified.

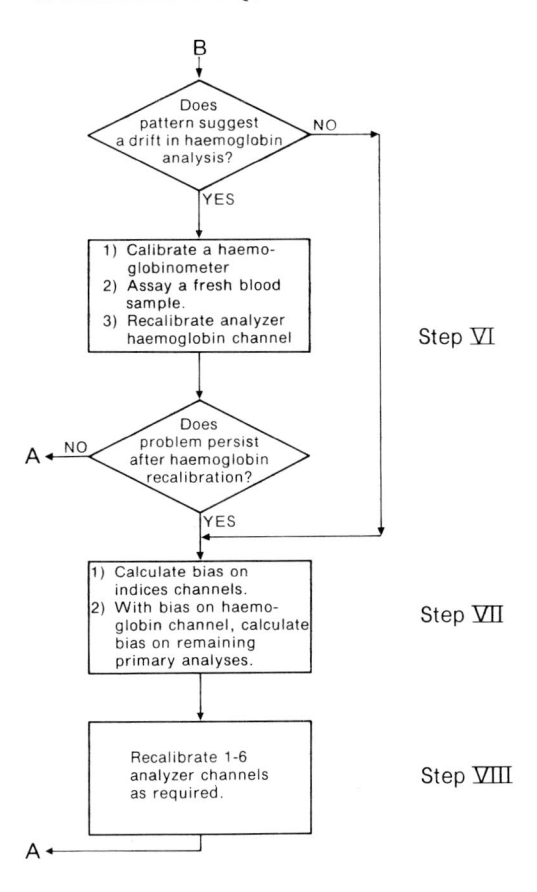

```
                              B
                              ↓
                    ┌───────────────────┐
                    │  Does pattern     │   NO
                    │  suggest a drift  │──────→
                    │  in haemoglobin   │
                    │  analysis?        │
                    └───────────────────┘
                              │ YES
                              ↓
              ┌─────────────────────────────┐
              │ 1) Calibrate a haemo-       │
              │    globinometer             │
              │ 2) Assay a fresh blood      │     Step VI
              │    sample.                  │
              │ 3) Recalibrate analyzer     │
              │    haemoglobin channel      │
              └─────────────────────────────┘
                              │
                              ↓
                    ┌───────────────────┐
              NO    │  Does problem     │
         A ←───────│  persist after    │
                    │  haemoglobin      │
                    │  recalibration?   │
                    └───────────────────┘
                              │ YES
                              ↓
              ┌─────────────────────────────┐
              │ 1) Calculate bias on        │
              │    indices channels.        │
              │ 2) With bias on haemo-      │     Step VII
              │    globin channel, calculate│
              │    bias on remaining        │
              │    primary analyses.        │
              └─────────────────────────────┘
                              │
                              ↓
              ┌─────────────────────────────┐
              │ Recalibrate 1-6             │
              │ analyzer channels           │     Step VIII
              │ as required.                │
              └─────────────────────────────┘
                              │
         A ←─────────────────┘
```

Fig. 7.1 (cont'd)

Step IV: determine the quantitative significance of any observed bias

Any differences between the observed means and the target mean indices must first be evaluated for quantitative significance. Clearly, any deviations below some threshold should be ignored since unnecessary attempts to recalibrate the analyzer will be detrimental rather than helpful to quality control. The decision as to appropriate threshold levels depends both upon the analyzer that is being used and upon the clinical significance of the changes. It is impractical to attempt any changes that are smaller than the smallest step to which the analyzer can respond. It is likewise of little use to attempt recalibration if the bias is well below clinically detectable limits. For most analyzers and on most channels no recalibration should be attempted until the bias is well over 2 per cent and has persisted through at least two consecutive patient data batches.

Step V: determine if the change is real or artefactual

A slow change in one or more of the indices that persists over several data batches causes few problems in interpretation: there is loss of calibration in the channels which have changed. Abrupt shifts in the range of 3 to 5 per cent that

134 QUALITY CONTROL

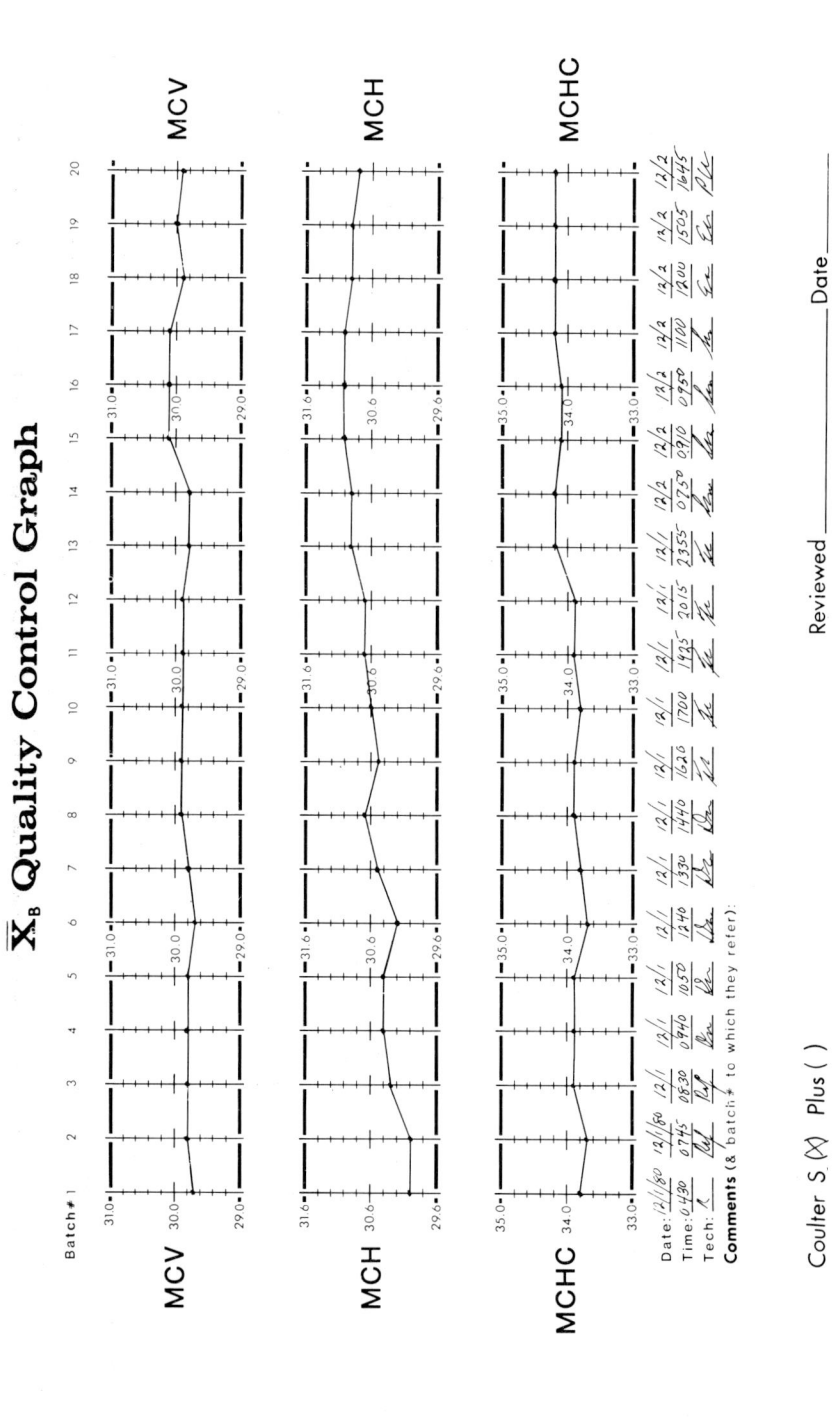

Fig. 7.2 Quality control based on patients' data. As the mean indices are computed they are entered under the appropriate batch number. Pattern recognition is enhanced if consecutive data points are joined and the MCV results are divided by 3 prior to plotting.

occur without warning between one data batch and the next are more difficult to interpret. Has the analyzer suffered a mechanical or electronic malfunction that represents a real loss of calibration and which will affect all subsequent analyses? If so, immediate recalibration is required. The other possibility is that a mistake in data entry or a non-random sequence of patient samples is responsible. If this latter possibility is the cause, then no action is required since the data from the next n patients when calculated will show the analyzer to be still correctly calibrated. The quickest road to verification is the re-analysis of any of the blood samples previously analyzed at a time when all of the observed indices were acceptably close to the target means. If the analyzer has truly lost calibration, the repeat analyses will fail to agree with the results previously obtained on that particular specimen. The channels that are incorrectly calibrated will be pinpointed by the differences.

A simpler and more pragmatic approach is simply to do nothing, particularly if a new batch of data will be forthcoming shortly. It is unusual for an analyzer to lose calibration abruptly. When it does so through mechanical or electronic failure, the calibration loss is unlikely to be less than 5 per cent. Consequently, most of the time, when an apparent calibration loss appears abruptly between one data batch and the next, it represents an artefact rather than a real loss of calibration. Once again, it must be emphasized that it is important to minimize or eliminate manual data entry errors and to ensure that the presentation of patient samples to the analyzer is truly random. These two causes account for virtually all of the episodes of artefactual calibration loss.

Step VI: calculate the bias present in the six RBC parameters
Once the differences between the observed and the target mean values have been accepted as both quantitatively significant and indicative of real calibration loss, the adjustments required in each of the six red cell related, analytical channels should be calculated. In order to perform this calculation one more data item is required — the bias present in any one of the primary measurements. For reasons already discussed the primary measurement usually chosen for this purpose is the measurement of hemoglobin. While the process of checking the calibration of the hemoglobin channel will be routinely performed at preset intervals, the data from this process is necessary for the performance of Step VI and for that reason will be discussed here.

Calibration of the hemoglobin assay channel
A hemoglobinometer and a diluent that meets the specifications of a national[7] or international reference body such as the NCCLS Standard: TSH-15, Reference Procedure for the Quantitative Determination of Hemoglobin in blood, should be used. These specifications, in brief, require the use of a Drabkins-type diluent (see Ch 2).

A certified standard solution of cynamethemoglobin should be purchased for use in the calibration of a suitable spectrophotometer or hemoglobinometer. Erlenmeyer flasks or suitably large test tubes and Class A pipettes comprise the rest of the equipment required. A full standard curve, constructed after the procedure described in the NCCLS Standard, needs to be constructed only at quarterly intervals and after major adjustments or bulb replacement on the spectrophotometer or colorimeter.

Three fresh, whole blood samples should be analyzed in duplicate for their hemoglobin content on the recently calibrated hemoglobinometer (or spectrophotometer). Analysis of these same blood samples on the whole blood analyzer (also in duplicate) will permit the calculation of a per cent bias factor for each sample and an average for all three. If the average bias amounts to more than 2 per cent, then the hemoglobin channel on the whole blood analyzer should be recalibrated and the three whole blood samples reanalyzed. Because it may be necessary to run each sample through the whole blood analyzer more than once, it is wise to initially choose samples that contain sufficient blood for repeat analyses. Several runs on the whole blood analyzer in addition to the analysis on the hemoglobinometer may be necessary.

At least once a month it is important to verify the linearity of the hemoglobin assay by manipulation of the red cell/plasma ratio of a whole blood sample so as to provide aliquots with hemoglobin values that cover the clinially encountered range. The hemoglobin values expected can be determined by performing packed cell volume determinations on the original sample and on all of the diluted/concentrated aliquots.

Once the bias (or absence of bias) of the hemoglobin channel has been determined, the bias of the red cell count and of the hematocrit can be calculated by means of the appropriate formulas.

$$RBC_{bias} = Hb_{bias}/MCH_{bias}$$
$$PCV_{bias} = Hb_{bias}/MCHC_{bias}$$

This latter equation takes a different form for those analyzers (i.e. Coulter®) which measure MCV rather than PCV:

$$PCV_{bias} = MCV_{bias} \times RBC_{bias}$$

It is convenient to calculate the bias as a percentage plus or minus, so as to indicate the appropriate adjustment to be made in each of the channels. At the conclusion of this process, the bias in all six of the red cell related parameters has been either measured directly or has been calculated.

Step VII: recalibrate one to six channels as required

The recalibration process will be unique to the whole blood analyzer that is being monitored. Typically it will require the manual adjustment of a series of potentiometers. It is important to maintain a before-and-after record of the potentiometer settings in the quality control record by noting the percentage change in each of the channels that were recalibrated. If the whole blood analyzer permits a direct digital entry of the per cent bias adjustment, the process is considerably simpler. After each recalibration, the analyzer must be watched closely for at least the time required to accumulate and calculate two patient data batches. This information will make it possible to verify that the appropriate channels were modified by the right amount and in the right direction.

This completes the recalibration process. The routine now returns to Step II awaiting the input of another batch of n patients. In the normal course of events the daily quality control routine will involve only the performance of Steps II and III. Analyzer recalibration should be necessary only at intervals of days to weeks; only then will the execution of Steps IV through VIII be necessary.

PATTERN INTERPRETATION — IDENTIFYING THE PROBLEM

As the quality control data plots are followed, a series of patterns will be recognized. Each pattern is specific for a particular analyzer and for a particular type of calibration loss. A list of all of the possible patterns would be an unwieldy and relatively useless document for two reasons. First, many of the possible patterns require such a fortuitous juxtaposition of qualitatively similar changes in independent measurements that they are rarely, if ever, encountered in real life. Second, such a listing is analyzer-specific since it depends upon the way in which the various pieces of input information are combined to produce the output — the six red cell related measurements.

The magnitude of the task can be better appreciated by considering the underlying mathematics. Three indices are being monitored and each may be running high, low or normal (above, below or on the population mean value). There are thus 3^3 or 27 combinations possible. By far, the commonest calibration failure will result from drift in only a single one of the primary measurements (these are usually the PCV, RBC and Hb). Since each of the red cell indices utilizes two of these three primary measurements, there will always be one of the indices that is unaffected. If we limit consideration to those cases in which two indices change and one remains stable, the number of possible patterns drops from 27 to 12. Of the 12 patterns which are theoretically possible only six occur because the relationships between the indices and the primary determinations are fixed. The Hb, for instance, is in the numerator of both the MCH and the MCHC calculation. Clearly, any pattern which results from drift in the Hb determination will show the MCH and the MCHC changing in the same direction. Both for illustrative purposes and because these six patterns are going to be frequently seen, the process of identifying them will be explained in some detail. A clear understanding of how the patterns originate on any one analyzer will make it easier for the user to identify unusual patterns on similar

Table 7.2 Patterns of change in the red cell indicies of patients samples as a result of changes in the measurement of Hb, RBC and PCV.

Index	Packed cell volume Increased	Packed cell volume Decreased	Red cell count Increased	Red cell count Decreased	Hemoglobin Increased	Hemoglobin Decreased	Index Derivation
MCV	High	Low	Low	High	Normal	Normal	$\dfrac{PCV}{RBC}$
MCH	Normal	Normal	Low	High	High	Low	$\dfrac{Hb}{RBC}$
MCHC	Low	High	Normal	Normal	High	Low	$\dfrac{Hb}{PCV}$

analyzers. It will also make it possible for each user to tabulate the possible patterns on a new and unfamiliar instrument.

A simple way of tabulating the six common patterns is illustrated in Table 7.2. The analyzer used here for illustrative purposes derives its output in the classical fashion by measuring the packed cell volume, the red cell count and the hemoglobin of a blood sample. It then calculates the indices in the usual manner. To utilize the Table the various patterns encountered are first located in the body of the table. The defect responsible can then be identified by reading up to the column heading. Both for the patterns listed in this Table and for those seen more rarely the first attempt at identification should be inspection of the equation by which the index is calculated. For this reason the index derivations are listed in the final column of both this Table and in Table 7.3.

All of the patterns listed above are unique — each is characteristic of an increase or decrease in a particular primary analytical module. In the case of a commonly used series of whole blood analyzers — the Coulter S, Sr and Plus — the patterns are, unfortunately, not so clear cut. These machines do not measure packed cell volume directly. The MCV is measured and the PCV is calculated from the MCV and the RBC. As a consequence, the MCV appears both in the listings of primary measurements and as one of the indices. This limits the

Table 7.3 Patterns of change in the red cell indices of patients samples which are characteristic of a shift in calibration of one of the analytical modules of the Coulter whole blood analyzer.

Index	Mean cell volume Increased	Decreased	Red cell count Increased	Decreased	Hemoglobin Increased	Decreased	Index Derivation
MCV	High	Low	Normal	Normal	Normal	Normal	MCV
MCH	Normal	Normal	Low	High	High	Low	$\dfrac{Hb}{RBC}$
MCHC	Low	High	Low	High	High	Low	$\dfrac{Hb}{RBC \times MCV}$

uniqueness of the Coulter® patterns. As can be seen from Table 7.3, the patterns for an increase in the RBC and a decrease in the Hb measurement are indistinguishable. Likewise, the patterns which result from a decrease in the RBC and an increase in the Hb are identical. This does not cause as severe a problem as might be anticipated because the hemoglobin analysis is calibrated against a primary standard and can be readily rechecked if in question. Information about the presence or absence of bias on the hemoglobin channel enables the ambiguity of the patterns to be clarified.

The Coulter® Counter whole blood analyzer has been the instrument most frequently controlled by the use of patients' data. As a consequence, more is known about the patterns characteristic of various malfunctions of this machine and some of these patterns have been described.[8,9,10] It is instructive to correlate several of the more common patterns with the underlying analyzer problem as a general exercise in troubleshooting whole blood analyzers.

MCH and MCHC elevated (Fig. 7.3, Batches 1 to 10)
From Table 7.3 the cause for simultaneous changes in these two indices is iden-

$\overline{X}_B$ Quality Control Graph

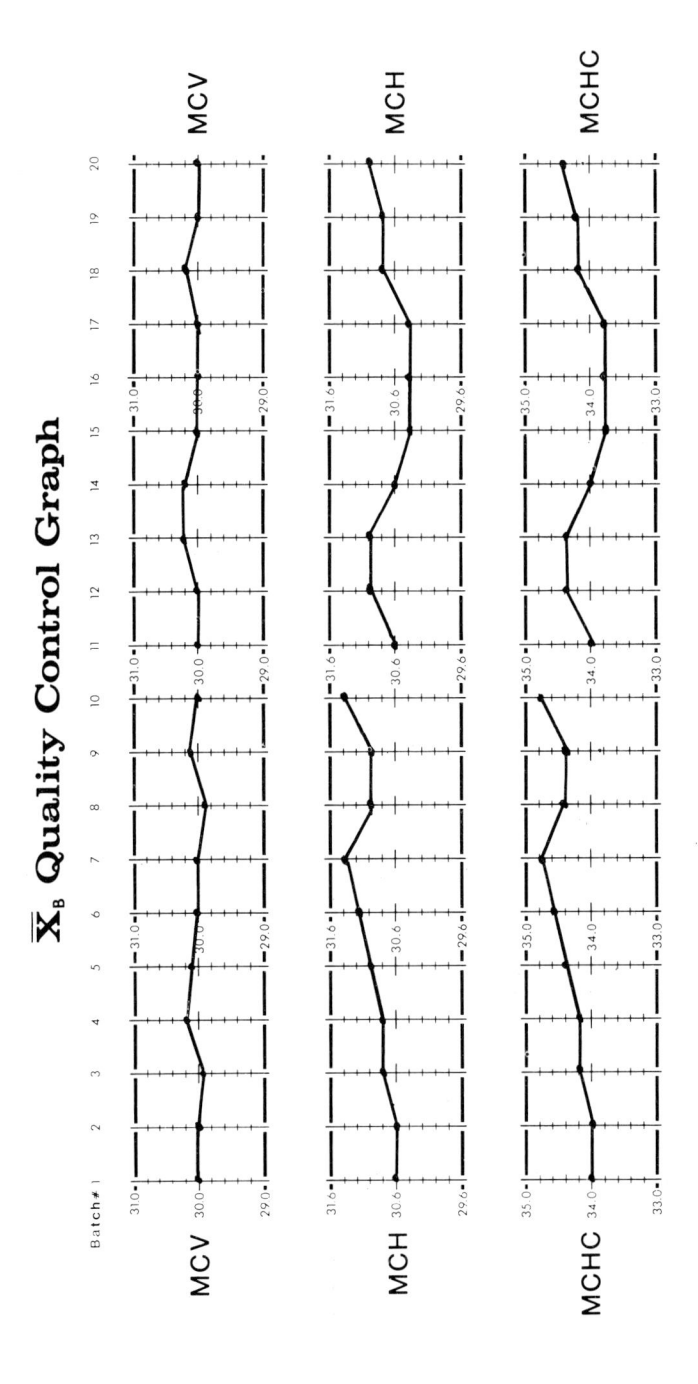

Fig. 7.3 Quality control based on patients' data; changes in MCH and MCHC caused by changes in RBC and Hb.

$\overline{X}_B$ Quality Control Graph

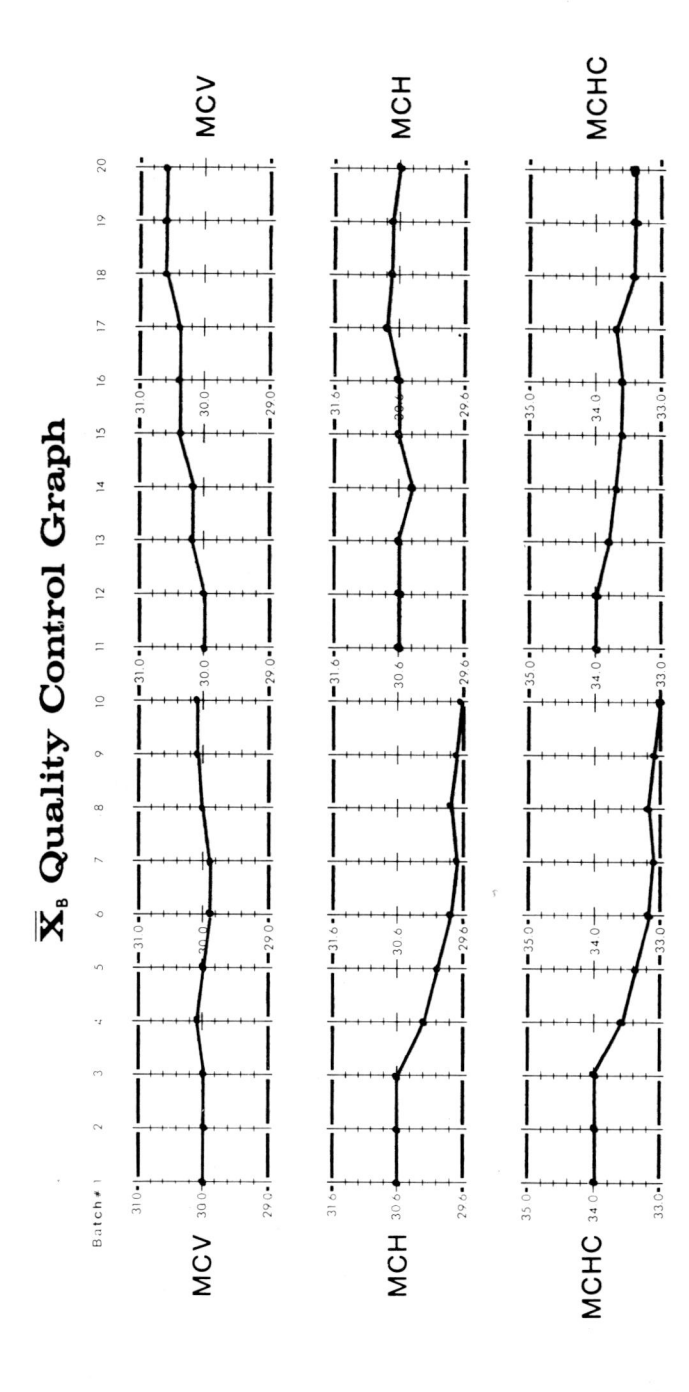

Fig. 7.4 Quality control based on patients' data; changes in MCV, MCH and MCHC caused by incorrect replacement of Hb light bar (Batches 1–10) and incorrect location of aperture tubes (Batches 11–20).

tified as a change in the RBC or Hb. If the Hb standardization is correct, the cause will frequently be traced to a malfunction of the sampling valve. If this valve fails to cycle completely when making the second dilution of a blood sample for the RBC count then the RBC will fall. This will produce a characteristic simultaneous elevation of MCH and MCHC. The MCV will, of course, be unaffected.

MCH and MCHC show fluctuating changes (Fig. 7.3, Batches 11 to 20)
As already noted, on the Coulter®, this means either a Hb or an RBC miscalibration. Hydraulic malfunction will not infrequently cause an erroneous Hb result. If the transfer of the lysed and diluted Hb containing solution is not complete, then major problems with carryover will ensue. The pattern of the patient data will show fluctuating, simultaneous changes in MCH and MCHC.

MCH and MCHC decreased (Fig. 7.4, Batches 1 to 10)
If, after maintenance procedures have been carried out, the hemoglobin light bar is not properly reseated, the hemoglobin value will fall and so will the MCH and MCHC.

MCV elevated and MCHC low (Fig. 7.4, Batches 11 to 20)
The cause for this pattern is a calibration loss in the MCV analytical module (Table 7.3). A relatively frequent cause of such a loss is a misalignment of the aperture tubes in the baths. If the tubes are placed too close to the walls of the counting baths the flow conditions through the orifices are affected. This in turn affects the MCV and produces a characteristic change in the MCV of the patient data.

The remaining Coulter® patterns fall into two groups. One is composed of those patterns in which only one index is affected; these are usually due to an arithmetic error in the calculation of that index. The patterns in the other group are those which show an increase or a decrease in two of the three indices, but which could only be caused by simultaneous opposite changes of approximately equal magnitudes in two of the primary measurements. For obvious reasons, patterns in this second category are unusual — except for one!

MCV and MCH synchronous elevation (Fig. 7.5 Batches 1 to 10)
This is probably the most common change seen in Coulter® S and Ssr analyzers. Since it can only be caused by an increase in the MCV accompanied by a simultaneous decrease of equal magnitude in the RBC (Table 7.4) an adequate cause for this unlikely juxtaposition must be sought. The red cell counting apertures are a common link between the two analyses. Protein buildup on these apertures decreases the RBC count. Simultaneously, because the apertures are now smaller, the red cells traversing them occupy a greater proportion of the aperture and appear larger. The result is a simultaneous rise in both MCV and MCH values.

MCV, MCH and particularly MCHC elevation (Fig. 7.5, Batches 11 to 20)
For good measure there is an unusual pattern sometimes encountered in which

142 QUALITY CONTROL

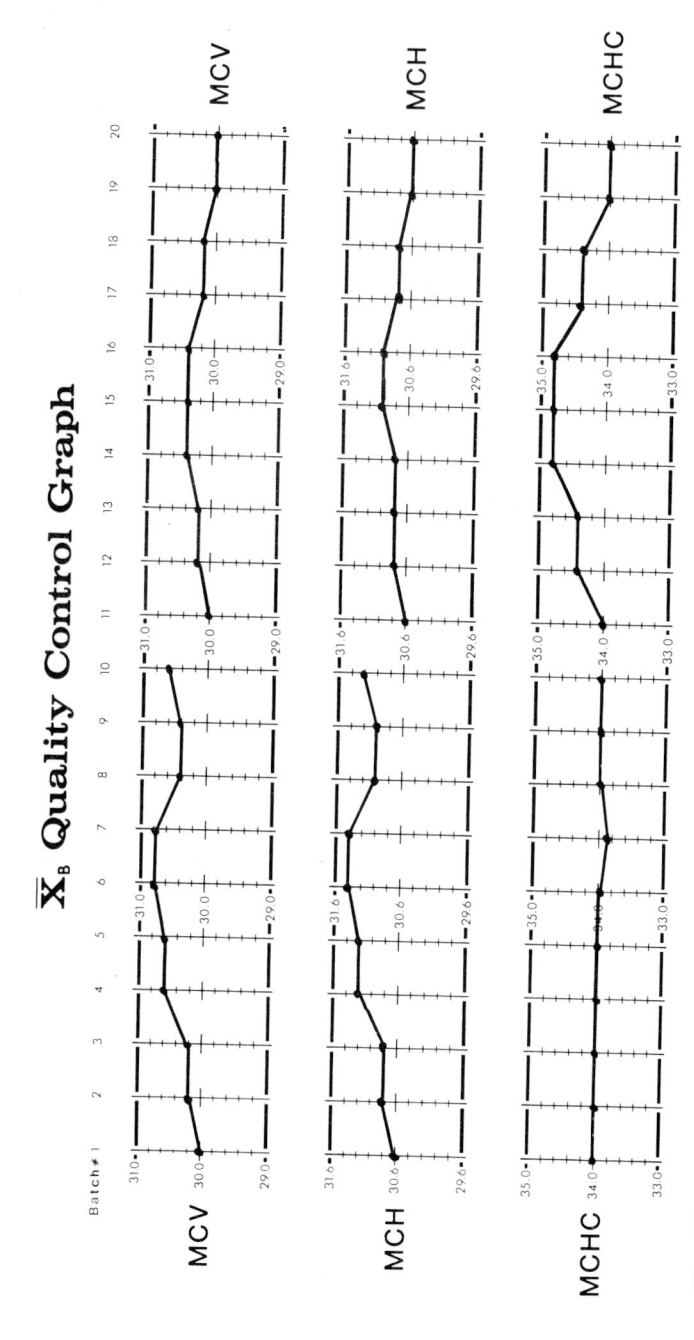

$\overline{X}_B$ Quality Control Graph

Fig. 7.5 Quality control based on patients data; synchronous changes in MCV & MCH caused by aperture narrowing (Batches 1–10) and synchronous changes in MCV, MCH and MCHC caused by bubbles (Batches 11–20)

Table 7.4 Patterns of change in the red cell indices of patients samples as a result of simultaneous but oppposite changes in the measurement of the MCV and RBC by the Coulter® whole blood analyzer.

Index	Mean cell volume Increased	Decreased
MCV	High	Low
MCH	High	Low
MCHC	Normal	Normal
	Decreased	Increased
	Red cell count	

all three indices rise but in which the MCHC rises twice as much as the other two. This come about when a defect in the analyzer pneumatic system permits large numbers of cell sized bubbles to remain in the counting chambers long enough to be counted.

APPENDIX

This appendix consists of a portfolio of log sheets. They illustrate the various records which have proven useful over a seven year period in a large hematology laboratory which has relied exclusively upon patients' data for quality control purposes during that time. The record formats shown were all designed for use with a specific selection of instruments. The whole blood analyzer was a Coulter® S; the hemoglobinometer/colorimeter was a modified Klett, the digital particle counter was a Coulter® ZBI. A different whole blood analyzer backed up by a different hemoglobinometer and an alternative, reference, red cell counter would require modifications in several of the formats. The modifications are likely to be minor and the principles exemplified by the records will apply to any selection of instruments presently capable of supporting a quality control program based on patients' data.

Figure 7.A1

Calibration verification log for white blood cell counts. Checking the set point of the WBC analyzer module is an integral part of the daily quality control program. A more extensive procedure performed in triplicate as described by Gilmer et al[4] should be performed for primary calibration.

While it is possible to determine the true mean WBC for the patient population and then to use this value as a target mean against which to compare the observed means derived from N patients, this approach is not as useful in this circumstance as it is for the red cell related measurements. The biological

QUALITY CONTROL

Calibration Verification Log — White Cell Count

Date	Tech	Acc No	COULTER Count 1 (Wash)	COULTER Count 2 (A)	BG	ZBI Count 1	ZBI Count 2	Ave (B)	$\frac{A}{B}$ (%)	Supervisor and Comments
1										
2										
3										
4										
5										
6										
7										
8										
9										
10										
11										
12										
13										
14										
15										
16										
17										
18										
19										
20										
21										
22										
23										
24										
25										
26										
27										
28										
29										
30										
31										

Coulter S ( )   Plus ( )   Reviewed_____ Date_____

Fig. 7.A1

variability of the WBC in a patient population is so much larger than that of the red cell indices (CV in the order of 60 per cent for the WBC compared to about 6 per cent for the red cell indices) that the quantity of patient data required is unacceptably large for routine clinical application. As a consequence, the WBC is calibrated daily against a reference method, in this case a dual threshold, digital particle counter, the Coulter ZBI.

The WBC of a single, fresh, whole blood sample is measured on the whole blood analyzer. The specimen should be run through twice to eliminate any carryover. A result from the first run is entered into the record as Count 1 (Wash). The second count (A) is used in the subsequent calculations. The same blood sample is then diluted 1:50 with an isotonic diluent using Class A glassware. The red cells in the diluted sample are lysed with Zapoglobin®. The background count on the reference cell counting instrument is measured followed by duplicate counts on the diluted sample. The mean of these duplicate results is calculated and the difference between this and the background count corrected for dilution to give the ZBI white cell count (B). The second count obtained on the whole blood analyzer is then expressed as a per cent of the mean count (B) obtained from the reference procedure. The result is recorded under heading 'A/B' and should remain at 100 ± 3 per cent.

Figure 7.A2
Calibration verification log for hemoglobin. This is a record of the information which accompanies each verification or recalibration of the hemoglobin determination.

One of the primary determinations must be standardized against reference methodology if the approach to quality control based on patient's data is to be implemented correctly. Because of the ready availability of stable cyanmethemoglobin solutions of certified hemoglobin content, the hemoglobin analysis is the measurement usually chosen. This process does not need to be repeated every day. If the analyzer is stable and the plot of the indices shows no change in calibration of more than 1.5 per cent it is sufficient to recheck the calibration of this analytical module once or twice a week. There is a small chance that a deviation in the hemoglobin module will be exactly balanced by a similar deviation in the RBC. Under these circumstances both would go unnoticed until the next hemoglobin recalibration. The chances that these two primary determinations will drift simultaneously in similar directions and that the deviations will be of similar magnitude are vanishingly small. It would appear to be unnecessary to protect against this eventuality by increasing the frequency of hemoglobin recalibration.

For recalibration three fresh whole blood samples are analyzed in duplicate on the Coulter® whole blood analyzer. Duplicate manual 1:251 dilutions of the same samples are then made using Class A glassware and the modified Drabkins diluent specified in the NCCLS standard TSH-15. The absorbance of each dilution and of duplicates of a cyanmethemoglobin standard are measured on the hemoglobinometer and the mean absorbances calculated. From these data the hemoglobin content of the patients samples is calculated. The bias present in the hemoglobin channel of the whole blood analyzer is then expressed as a per-

Calibration verification log: hemoglobin

Date	Tech Spvr	Acc No.	COULTER Hb 1 (Wash)	COULTER Hb 2 (A)	SPECTROPHOTOMETER/HEMOGLOBINOMETER Absorbance 1	Absorbance 2	Mean	CALCULATIONS	$\frac{A}{B}$ (%)	Cyamethemoglobin Standard
		Std						$\text{Mean}_n \times \frac{\text{Assay}}{\text{Mean Std}} \times \frac{251}{100} = \text{Hb (B)}$		Brand: Lot No: Exp date: Assay: Sens. ratio.5/5
		Std						$\text{Mean}_n \times \frac{\text{Assay}}{\text{Mean Std}} \times \frac{251}{100} = \text{Hb (B)}$		Brand: Lot No: Exp date: Assay: Sens. ratio.5/5
		Std						$\text{Mean}_n \times \frac{\text{Assay}}{\text{Mean Std}} \times \frac{251}{100} = \text{Hb (B)}$		Brand: Lot No: Exp date: Assay: Sens. ratio.5/5
		Std						$\text{Mean}_n \times \frac{\text{Assay}}{\text{Mean Std}} \times \frac{251}{100} = \text{Hb (B)}$		Brand: Lot No: Exp date: Assay: Sens. ratio.5/5
		Std						$\text{Mean}_n \times \frac{\text{Assay}}{\text{Mean Std}} \times \frac{251}{100} = \text{Hb (B)}$		Brand: Lot No: Exp date: Assay: Sens. ratio.5/5

Coulter S [ ]   Plus [ ]   Reviewed_____ Date_____

Fig. 7.A2

INTRALABORATORY QUALITY CONTROL USING PATIENTS' DATA 147

Fig. 7.A3 Coulter S Daily Maintenance Log

148 QUALITY CONTROL

Fig. 7.A4 Coulter S Daily Electronics Log

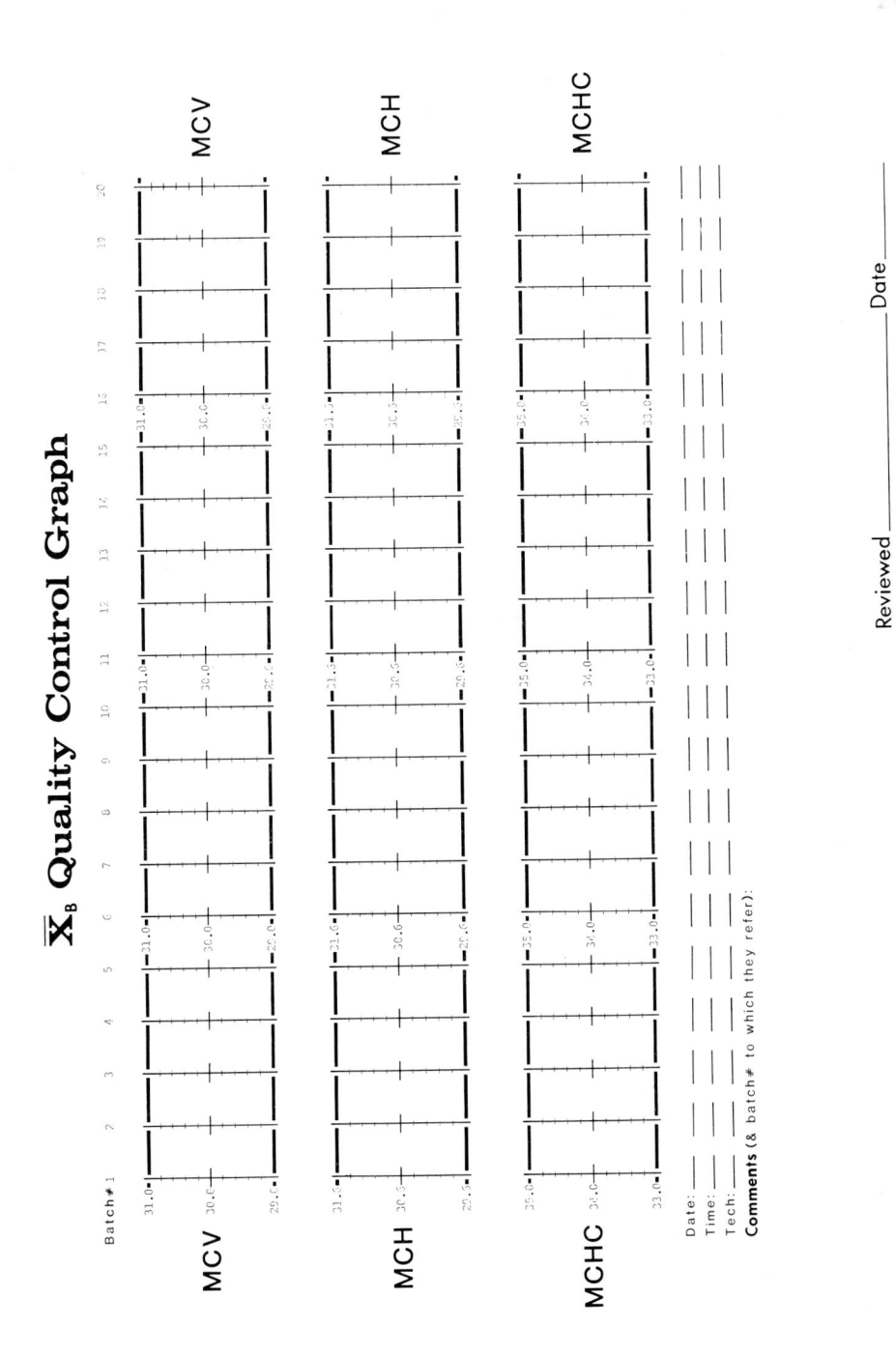

INTRALABORATORY QUALITY CONTROL USING PATIENTS' DATA 149

$\overline{X}_B$ Quality Control Graph

Fig. 7.A5

centage of the result obtained by the reference method compared with that from the analyzer for the same sample.

Figures 7.A3 and 7.A4
Forms for recording various machine parameters for daily quality control purposes.

Regardless of the methods used to maintain correct analyzer calibration it is advisable routinely to record the background counts on both WBC and RBC apertures. It is also wise to measure and record the voltages as well as the vacuum and air pressure levels at various specified check points throughout the analyzer. With this data available the process of locating a malfunction in the whole blood analyzer is simplified. It is even more useful coupled with the premonitory instability in the quality control of the patients' data. Unexplained cyclical variations or increasing instability in the plots of the mean red cell indices will often herald a mechanical failure of the analyzer by hours or days. Experienced observers can then prepare for the impending breakdown by readying backup equipment and alerting the service bureau.

Figure 7.A5
A format for quality control based on $\overline{X}_B$. The MCV should be divided by 3 before it is plottted. Pattern recognition is enhanced if consecutive data points are joined by straight lines. Each entry should be initialled by the person responsible for evaluating the data.

REFERENCES

1. Bull B, Elashoff R M 1974 The use of patient-derived hematology data in quality control. Proceedings of the San Diego Biomedical Symposium 13: 515–519
2. Bull B S 1980 Quality control based on statistical analysis of complete blood count data. R M Schmidt, section editor, CRC Handbook of Clinical Laboratory Science 2: 405–408
3. Bull B S, Elashoff R M, Heilbron D C, Couperus J 1974 A study of various estimators for the derivation of quality control procedures from patient erythrocyte indices. American Journal of Clinical Pathology 61: 473–481
4. Gilmer P R, Williams L J, Koepke J A, Bull B S 1977 Calibration methods for automated hematology instruments. American Journal of Clinical Pathology 68: 185–194
5. Model 970, Royco Instruments, 1032 Elwell Court, Palo Alto CA 94303
6. Korpman R A, Bull B S 1976 The implementation of a robust estimator of the mean for quality control on a programmable calculator or laboratory computer. American Journal of Clinical Pathology 65: 252–253
7. Reference procedure for the quantitative determination of hemoglobin in blood TSH — 15, NCCLS, 771 E. Lancaster Avenue, Villanova PA 19085
8. Bull B S 1975 A statistical approach to quality control. In: Lewis S M, Coster J F (eds) Quality control in haematology. Academic Press, London, P 111–122
9. Koepke J A, Protexter T J 1980 Quality assurance: producing continuously useful hematology data. Lab World, February: 21–28
10. Koepke J A, Protexter T J 1981 Quality assurance for multichannel hematology instruments. Four years experience with patient mean erythrocyte indices. American Journal of Clinical Pathology 75: 28–33

8
Intralaboratory Quality Control Using Control Samples

C. Ricketts

INTRODUCTION

The need for an effective system of statistical quality control in the hematology laboratory has become apparent during the last two decades. Before that time the production of a result by the laboratory was the end of a process of painstaking effort and personal attention. The advent of automated equipment for the analysis of blood samples has radically changed the practice of laboratory hematology. No longer can the hematologist have the same confidence that each result leaving his laboratory is accurate because they are now being produced by a complex but rigid mechanical system rather than by competent, adaptable and responsible people. In addition, automation of laboratory methods has inevitably brought an explosive increase in the number of tests requested and the laboratory has come under increasing pressure. At this stage the introduction of an effective and efficient system of statistical quality control becomes essential for the laboratory if it is to continue to provide the excellent service expected of it.

Hematologists are not alone in their need for quality control: it has been an integral part of many other activities for some considerable time (see Ch. 1). Although we may be reluctant to admit a comparison between the laboratory and a production industry some degree of detachment will allow us to see a parallel. Much of the effort of a modern hematology laboratory is channeled towards the routine production of numerical results of a uniformly high standard. Similarly, a production industry aims to produce some product of a uniform quality; the quality of the product can usually be determined by the numerical value of some characteristic be it weight, diameter or tensile strength. When the quality of a product changes the industry may lose money and this has provided a considerable stimulus to the development of methods of statistical quality control in industry. As a result the principles, practice and statistical characteristics of methods of quality control have been well tried. Hematology is therefore in the fortunate position of being able to benefit from developments in other fields. Much of what is good in quality control can be directly applied in hematology while some practices may require modification. There is no need to re-invent the wheel: all that is required is to make it the right size.

The application of quality control to routine blood counting has hitherto been limited by the lack of a suitable preparation to serve as a whole blood control. Recent application of techniques for stabilizing and preserving whole blood[1] have resulted in the production of a stable whole blood control suitable for use with the Coulter S blood counter. When used in conjunction with appropriate statistical techniques[2] effective and efficient quality control can be achieved. This chapter will present methods for preparing a whole blood control, the means by which it may be used in the laboratory and the methods for analyzing the results to provide a single cohesive technique for quality control of automated blood counting.

The aim of intralaboratory quality control is to ensure that results from an individual laboratory are comparable from day to day and from year to year. The problems of interlaboratory quality control, ensuring that results from different laboratories are accurate or at least comparable, are discussed in Chapter 6. In the following two sections the use of control samples and the methods available for analyzing the data obtained will be discussed. The subsequent section is the heart of the chapter: it contains the detailed methodology for the application of quality control using control samples in the hematology laboratory. Following this, a method of automating the analysis of the data will be described. The emphasis will be exclusively on quality control of automatic blood counters. However, the principles and methods apply equally well to any other test procedure in hematology.

CONTROL SAMPLES

Quality control of a hematology test procedure is based on monitoring some aspects of the process to ensure that it is accurate, precise and performing in the same manner at all times. That is, if the same blood sample were analyzed time and again the same result (within the limits of experimental error) would be obtained on each occasion. However, the patients' samples which come into the laboratory may each be different and the hematological characteristics of the patient population may change from day to day.[3] Separate control samples must therefore be used.

A *control preparation* has an arbitrary but constant value for a particular constituent.[4] Its most important property is that it should be stable and the value for the constituent of interest should be constant over a long period. For most test procedures a stable period of about one month should be a practical minimum. The value of a constituent of a control preparation need not be specified: it can be determined by the test procedure after standardization. A constant test procedure will produce the same result each time a sample of the control preparation is analyzed. Any change in the results for the control samples will indicate a change in the test process. This is the principle which underlies the use of control samples for quality control. A *standard preparation* is distinguished from a control by having a specified and constant value for a particular constituent. Such standards include the international cyanmethemoglobin standard[6] or the standard solution described by the ICSH[7] for the determination of serum iron. There is no standard preparation of whole blood which may be used for the calibration and standardization of blood counters. The problem of standardization and methods of calibrating blood counters are described in

Chapter 2 and for the purposes of this chapter it is assumed that appropriate calibration has been carried out. The object is to detect any deviation from that condition so that it may be corrected before there is any clinically significant change in the accuracy of the results that are issued by the laboratory.

A major factor limiting the application of appropriate statistical techniques to automated blood counting has been the lack of a suitable stabilized whole blood control. Morgan et al[1] have described a newly developed preparation which fills this gap. The whole blood control consists of human red cells partially fixed with glutaraldehyde and chicken red cells fixed with formalin as a human white cell analogue. These cells are suspended in a synthetic medium containing antibiotics. An intensive study of the properties of this preparation has shown that, following an initial stabilization period of three to four weeks, the parameters of the whole blood remain stable for at least a further two months. The method of preparation has been published[5] but permission to use the method must be obtained in advance from the patent holder. A large hematology department may keep itself supplied with this control blood relatively easily. Alternatively, a group of laboratories could arrange for one of them to regularly supply the whole group. In Wales, the Blood Transfusion Service now provides this control blood for every hematology laboratory in the region.

The frequency with which control samples should be analyzed in the routine workflow of patients' samples is a matter for judgement and experience. Clearly, the more frequently control samples are analyzed the more rapidly will any faults be detected. Against this must be balanced the need to produce patients' results as rapidly as possible without allocating an excessive amount of the laboratory's resources to quality control. Experience suggests that a single control sample should be analyzed after approximately every 20 patients' samples. Provided that the quality control scheme is sufficiently sensitive to detect changes in a test procedure before they represent significant clinical changes this sampling frequency will provide an adequate degree of confidence. In some circumstances, such as when a test procedure is suspected of being unstable, it may be advisable to analyze the control preparation more frequently.

ANALYZING CONTROL RESULTS

The results from control samples provide an indication of the performance of the test procedure. Not only do they provide evidence of changes but, more importantly, they also give a positive indication when all is well. The analytical method must allow the laboratory to detect relatively small changes both rapidly and with confidence. There are two types of changes which can occur: a change in accuracy and a change in precision. When the process is performing properly then the results from control samples will be clustered about their mean value. A change in *accuracy* occurs when the mean value changes so that each result is now altered by a fixed amount. A change in *precision* occurs when the results remain distributed about their established mean value but they are less closely clustered. These different types of change are illustrated in Figure 8.1. The detection of changes in accuracy is relatively simple and well estab-

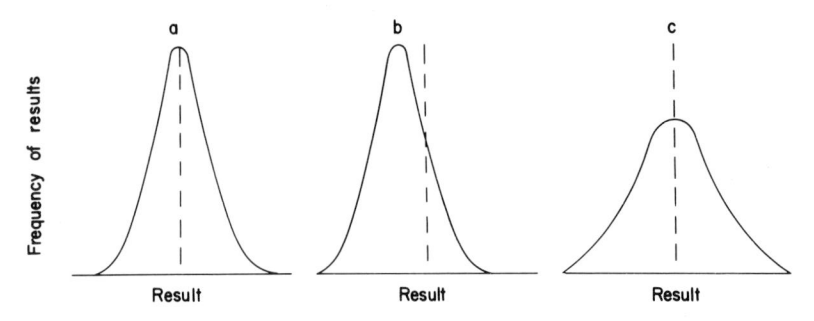

Fig. 8.1 The distribution of control sample results (a) when the test process is working normally, (b) when there is a change in accuracy, (c) when there is a change in precision. The dashed line shows the established process mean.

lished: changes in precision are more difficult to detect and have only recently received detailed attention. Methods for detecting changes in accuracy will be described first: changes in precision will be considered separately.

CHANGES IN ACCURACY

Control charts

A simple method of examining control results to detect a change in accuracy is to plot a graph of the result against the sample number (Ch. 1). The Shewhart control chart has two drawbacks. Only the current result, or at most the last two results, contributes towards an indication that there has been a change in accuracy. All the previous data, which contain some information about the performance of the test procedure, remains unused. In addition, the method makes no use of the values which fall within the limits but which may indicate a significant and consistent, albeit small, change. Both these limitations reduce the sensitivity of the method and it has largely been superseded by the more sensitive cumulative sum techniques.

Cumulative sum (cusum) techniques

Cusum graphs were originally developed to provide a greater visual impact than plotting control results: statistical techniques for analyzing cusum data evolved somewhat later. In cumulative sum techniques changes are detected using the cumulative sum of the differences between the test results and a reference or target value. That is, if the individual result of the ith control sample is x_i and the reference is m, the cusum after n control samples is $S_n = \sum_{i=1}^{n} (x_i - m)$.

There are two equivalent methods of assessing the cusum to detect a change in accuracy. The first method involves plotting a graph which gives a continuous picture of the test performance (Ch. 1) but in laboratory practice it can be somewhat time-consuming and tedious. For Normally distributed data a simple mask such as that described in Chapter 1 can be used to provide a rapid and exact assessment of the significance of changes in the slope of the cusum graph. The second, decision interval, method requires less calculation and no graph plotting and is readily carried out by a computer; however, it lacks the visual impact of a graph.

In a decision interval scheme an increase in the process mean may be detected by setting an upper reference value (URV) at m + k, where k is approximately half the minimum significant change which the laboratory wishes to detect. This is usually approximately one standard deviation of the methodological variability. As long as the control results are less than or equal to m + k no calculations are made. As soon as a control result exceeds the URV a cusum is started within m + k as the reference value. Thereafter it is the magnitude of this cusum which provides evidence of a change in accuracy. If the cusum exceeds a decision interval (DI), h, then a change in accuracy has occurred. Control results below the mean are analyzed in a similar way with a lower reference value (LRV) at m − k and a lower decision interval of −h. A typical laboratory worksheet for this type of control scheme for the Coulter S is shown in Figure 8.2.

Although the decision interval scheme might appear to be similar to the simple Shewhart control chart it is in fact directly equivalent to the cusum plot and mask. In this case the mask is the original 'V' from which that described in Chaper 1 is derived.[8] The two limbs of the V are inclined at an angle θ to the line OP of length d as shown in Figure 8.3. The V-mask is used by placing it on the cusum chart with the line OP horizontal and the point P coinciding with the last plotted point. If all the points of the graph are within the arms of the V then there has been no significant change in accuracy. If the cusum graph crosses either arm of the V then this indicates that there has been a change in accuracy and some corrective action must be taken. The characteristics of the control scheme, such as the size of changes in accuracy it will detect and how rapidly it will detect them, are determined by the values of d and θ.

As with the V-mask, the characteristics of the decision interval scheme are determined by the values of k and h. However, the method for choosing k and h can be shown to be the same as that for choosing d and θ.[9]

Consider a V-mask with parameters d and θ used on a cusum graph where the interval between points on the horizontal axis is equivalent to 2σ on the

Cusum control chart							Date:	
	Wbc		Rbc		Hb		MCV	
DI URV LRV								
Sample no.	Result	Cusum	Result	Cusum	Result	Cusum	Result	Cusum

Fig. 8.2 A laboratory worksheet for assessment of the cusum using a decision interval.

vertical axis: this is compared with a decision interval scheme with parameters k and h. The established mean is m. The decision interval will never indicate a change of accuracy while the difference between the control results and the mean is less than k. Similarly, the V-mask will never indicate a change if the slope of the cusum graph is less than the slope of the arms of the V-mask. Thus, for the decision interval scheme

$$|x_i - m| < k$$

and for the V-mask

$$\frac{|x_i - m|}{2\sigma} < \tan \theta$$

$$|x_i - m| < 2\sigma \tan \theta$$

Thus, if $k = 2\sigma \tan \theta$ these limitations are equivalent.

Now consider the point at which loss of control is indicated and, for simplicity, the case of an increase in the control results. The same argument applies to a decrease in the control result, but all expressions are then negative. For the decision interval scheme the sum of the differences $x_i - (m + k)$ must be greater than the decision interval

$$\Sigma [x_i - (m + k)] > h$$

By referring to Figure 8.2 and using a little geometry it can be seen that for the cusum graph to cross the V-mask

$$\sum_{B}^{A} [x_i - m] > PR = 2\sigma(d \tan \theta + s \tan \theta)$$

which can be expressed as

$$\sum_{B}^{A} [x_i - m - 2\sigma \tan \theta] > 2\sigma d \tan \theta$$

It is already established that $k = 2\sigma \tan \theta$ and so this expression becomes

$$\Sigma[x_i - (m + k)] > 2\sigma d \tan \theta$$

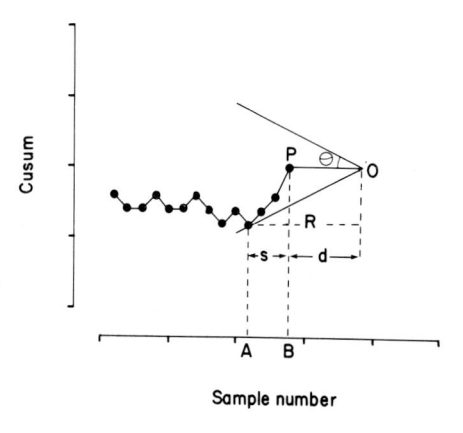

Fig. 8.3 Equivalence of decision rules for a cusum chart.

Thus the two schemes are equivalent when h = 2σd tan θ

To summarize, a V-mask scheme with parameters d and θ is equivalent to a decision interval scheme with parameters k and h when

$$k = 2\sigma \tan \theta$$
$$h = 2\sigma d \tan \theta$$

Therefore, the laboratory needs only to choose the performance of the control scheme to be able to specify equivalent V-mask and decision interval schemes.

Choosing the properties of a control scheme.
The hematologist should decide what properties he requires of a control scheme. This involves a decision of the size of change that requires to be detected, how rapidly it should be detected and what frequency of false positive indications is tolerable. The size of the change to be detected should be considered in the light of the known standard deviation of the test procedure and the clinical significance of a change of that magnitude in a patient's result. In general, it is useful to be able to detect calibration changes which do not represent clinically significant differences. The test procedure need not be expected to detect that change immediately but if it is consistent it should be detected within a few samples of it occurring. Larger changes would be detected more rapidly and smaller changes somewhat more slowly. It is equally important that the laboratory work should not be interrupted by too many indications of loss of accuracy when none has, in fact, occurred.

The size of change the laboratory requires to detect is usually expressed in terms of the process standard deviation σ. For most practical purposes the required change of y σ units in the mean should have a value of y between 1.5 and 4. When a change of y σ units has occurred the process should detect it within L_1 samples. This is called the average run length (ARL) when the test process has suffered a change of accuracy of that level. When no change has occurred the laboratory may expect a false positive warning once in every L_0 samples. This is the ARL when testing is in control. Cavill and Ricketts[2] have suggested that suitable values are y = 2, L_1 = 3, L_0 = 500. That is, the quality control scheme should be capable of detecting changes in the mean of two standard deviations within three samples but not expect a false indication of a change in accuracy more than once in every 500 control samples.

After choosing suitable values of y, L_1 and L_0 the parameters of the control scheme should be calculated. Ewan and Kemp[10] have presented nomograms for the derivation of k and h and Goldsmith and Whitfield[11] have calculated average run lengths of a variety of V-masks. Goldsmith and Whitfield[11] also developed two empirical formulae for calculating the ARLs of a control scheme from d and θ. These formulae can be used to determine the performance of any control scheme and also, by trial and error, to determine suitable values of d and θ (and hence k and h). These formulae are

$$\log_{10} \log_{10} L_0 = -0.5244 + 0.0398d + 1.1687 \tan \theta + 1.12641 \tan \theta \log d$$
$$L_1 = \frac{2d \tan \theta}{k - 2 \tan \theta} + \frac{2}{3}$$

For the average run lengths suggested by Cavill and Ricketts[2] the parameters of the control scheme are

d = 2.6, tan θ = ½
or h = 2.6σ, k = σ

SENSITIVITY OF QUALITY CONTROL TECHNIQUES

Cumulative sum techniques have been developed to provide a method of detecting small changes efficiently and effectively. However, the use of straightforward control charts (Shewhart charts) can be more effective at detecting large changes. Wetherill[9] provides an example of the relative average run lengths of both types of scheme with respect to the size of change. It would therefore seem appropriate to simultaneously run both cusum and control charts; however, this would produce a marked increase in the calculations involved, although automation may provide a solution. However, the control scheme described below is essentially the same as running the two schemes. Large deviations, such as those easily detected by control charts and which may be obscured by cusum charts, are rapidly detected.

When the cusum is zero any change greater than 3.6σ will produce a cusum greater than the decision interval and indicate loss of control. Similarly, two consecutive results more than 2.3σ from the mean will produce a cusum greater than the decision interval. It is when a positive cusum is running and a result below the lower reference value occurs that a large change may go undetected if a simple cusum scheme is in use. There is no clear theoretical rule as to how to proceed. An empirical approach is: if a cusum is running and changes sign, test the size of the deviation of the result from the current reference value. If this difference is greater than 2σ assume that some change has occurred. The rationale behind this argument is that, if a cusum is running there is some indication of a change: the reference value is not a bad measure of the current process mean. If a subsequent result lies further than 2σ from the reference value a large change in the current mean should be suspected.

The action to be taken in these circumstances is not to test the calibration but simply to change the frequency with which control samples are analyzed: three control samples are assayed consecutively and, if no loss of control is indicated, sampling proceeds as usual. Otherwise, the change is detected rapidly. Although this method is not exactly equivalent to the simultaneous use of a control chart and a cusum chart it does add some of the advantages of control charts to the cusum calculation.

CHANGES IN PRECISION

Techniques similar to those described above may be used to detect changes in precision. However, the application of cusum techniques to this problem is considerably less well understood. A major practical drawback of controlling precision is that additional control samples must be analyzed. While accuracy can be monitored by analyzing a single control sample on each occasion, the assessment of precision requires some measure of the spread of the results at each point. This requires a minimum of two samples to be analyzed on each occasion so that the spread can be estimated by the difference between the two results. The procedure becomes more sensitive as more samples are analyzed at each point but at a price. Even the use of two samples to monitor error doubles the quality control workload. Not only must an additional sample be analyzed but a second separate control chart must be constructed for monitoring precision. Whether this is worthwhile for many hematological tests is a matter for each hematologist to decide. If there is good reason to suppose that a particular test procedure is susceptible to a change in accuracy rather than a change in precision then it may be enough only to monitor accuracy. If, on the other hand, it is known that a test process is always accurate but may become unreliable as a result of a decrease in precision then it may be worthwhile monitoring precision alone. In a perfect world both accuracy and precision should be assessed. In most cases, however, resources may be limited and monitoring accuracy is probably more relevant. A change in accuracy may frequently be accompanied by a change in precision as a result of some malfunction and any remedial action should also improve precision.

As with the control of accuracy, where control charts or cusum techniques can be used, so it is with precision. These two methods will be discussed in turn. The use of control charts is well established and usually based on the range. The use of cusum techniques is a recent innovation and is best based on the variance.[12]

Control charts

The range of the samples tested on each occasion, that is the difference between the largest and smallest values obtained is plotted against the sample number. Action limits and warning limits can be used in the same way as for the control of accuracy although here it is the distribution of the range which is used to define these limits. The percentage points of the distribution of the range can be found in Pearson and Hartley.[13] It should be noted that the limits are not symmetrically placed about the mean range. For most purposes only a decrease in precision, which will produce an increase in the range, is of interest and only the upper limits need be drawn at an appropriate level.

Cumulative sum techniques

The use of cusum methods to monitor precision has been limited by the lack of formulae for calculating the parameters of a decision scheme and their average run length. However, recent developments by Rowlands[14] have provided suitable formulae. The technique has thus far been applied only to the control of radioimmunoassays but is easily transferred to any laboratory procedure. Wilson et al[12] have published average run lengths for a variety of V-masks when only two or three samples are analyzed on each occasion.

The control of precision can also be achieved using a decision interval scheme rather than a V-mask. The sample variance, s^2, is compared with the known variance of the test procedure, σ^2, by calculating s^2/σ^2. When the precision of the test procedure remains constant this ratio will fluctuate about 1. When the process becomes less precise s^2 will be greater than σ^2 and the ratio will be greater than 1. Similarly, any improvement in precision will produce values of s^2/σ^2 of less than 1. The target value for the variance ratio of any parameter is thus 1 and the deviation from this is given by $[(s^2/\sigma^2) - 1]$. The cumulative sum, S_n, of deviations of s^2/σ^2 is calculated:

$$S_n = \sum_{i=1}^{n}[(s_i^2/\sigma^2) - 1]$$

and plotted against the sample number.

The parameters of a V-mask for the assessment of changes in precision can be selected from Table 8.1 for the cases when either two or three samples are analyzed on each occasion. With these small sample numbers it is difficult to detect changes rapidly. For example, with two samples, if there is a change in the ratio of s/σ by a factor of two an average run length of six is required to detect this if the frequency of false positive indications is to be less than one in every three hundred. Considerably improvements are possible when the sample size is increased to three. In this case an average run length of four can be achieved with a frequency of false positive indications of less than one in 500.

Table 8.1 The characteristics of a V mask (d and θ) to detect a two fold change in variability of a process (S/σ ≥ 2) within a given number of control samples (L_1). The average run length before a false positive indication would be indicated is also given (L_2). (From Wilson et al 1980.[12])

		Number of replicate control samples				
		n = 2			n = 3	
L_1	d	θ	L_2	d	θ	L_2
4	4.36	17.98	51	6.40	22.97	559
5	7.79	16.13	128	9.03	22.76	2848
6	10.12	16.54	303	11.49	22.90	14357
7	12.92	16.35	701	—	—	—
8	15.46	16.43	1600	—	—	—
9	18.02	16.57	3624	—	—	—
10	20.57	16.50	8177	—	—	—

A METHOD OF QUALITY CONTROL

Statistical theory must be distilled into a practical system which can be applied in the hematology laboratory. The system that will be described is based on the practice in one laboratory: others may wish to vary some aspects of it by referring back to its theoretical basis which has been discussed in previous sections of this chapter. Application of such a system to the quality control of an automated test procedure consists of a number of different stages. These are:

A. Preparation of a suitable control material.
B. Calibration of the test procedure.
C. Establishing the mean and variance of the control in the test.
D. Analyzing the control samples in the test run.

E. Analyzing the control results and deciding whether a change has occurred.
F. Taking corrective action if a change has occurred.

This section will be limited to a description of quality control for the Coulter S blood counter. This is probably the most common item of automated equipment in hematology laboratories and accounts for more than half the results produced. Each of the stages which go to mke up a system of quality control will be described in turn.

The aim of this control scheme is to detect changes in the accuracy of the white cell count (Wbc) red cell count (Rbc), hemoglobin concentration (Hb) and mean corpuscular volume (MCV). The changes to be detected are such that they do not represent significant changes in a clinical result. For this reason they need not be detected at once but should be detected, on average, within three control samples of the change occurring. These changes are

Wbc $\pm 0.05 \times 10^9/1$
Rbc $\pm 0.10 \times 10^{12}/1$
Hb ± 0.2 g/dl
MCV ± 2 fl

The approach described here is based on the statistical analysis described previously but sprinkled with some empirical points which make for ease of practice in the laboratory.

A. PREPARATION OF WHOLE BLOOD CONTROL

A whole blood control suitable for use with the Coulter S has been described by Morgan et al[1] and details of its preparation have been published as a British Patent Specification,[5] and before using the process described below permission must be obtained from Mr R.A. Saunders, Scientific Adviser, Welsh Office, Pearl Assurance House, Greyfriars Road, Cardiff. The control material consists of stabilized human red cells and fixed chicken erythrocytes as an analogue of human white cells and is stable for at least two months. The preparation of the whole blood control can be divided into three separate processes. The chicken red cells must be fixed, the human red cells must be stabilized by partial fixation and then the two must be combined to produce a whole blood control. This 'recipe' is sufficient for 1 litre of control blood and should be scaled up to produce larger volumes. All materials and equipment must be sterile.

Preparation of fixed chicken red cells

1. 25 ml of fresh chicken blood is collected into heparinized acid-citrate-dextrose solution. Alternatively, 25 ml of adult chicken red cells suspended in an Alsever's solution are obtained from Tissue Culture Services Ltd., Slough, Bucks. In either case, centrifuge the cells and wash them three times in normal saline (0.9 per cent NaCl w/v) then resuspend the cells in their own volume of normal saline.

2. Nine volumes of neutral buffered saline solution are mixed with one volume of 400 g/l aqueous solution of formalin. Place 200 ml of this mixture in a 500 ml screw-topped container and heat to 37°C. Mix this on a magnetic stirrer and

slowly add the washed chicken red cells. Screw the top onto the container and continue to stir for five hours at 37°C. Then pour the cells in their suspending medium into centrifuge tubes and centrifuge at 500 g for five minutes. Remove the supernatant and wash at least three times with normal saline. It may be necessary to use a vortex mixer to resuspend the fixed cells between washes. Resuspend the cells in approximately twice their volume of phosphate buffered normal saline (ISOTON II, Coulter Electronics Ltd.) containing 0.1 g/l sodium azide. Mix and then store in a plastic bottle at 4°C.

Partial fixation of human red cells

3. Prepare 2 litres of a modified Alsever's solution as follows: add 38 g dextrose monohydrate, 8.4 g sodium chloride, 16 g trisodium citrate and 1 g citric acid to a 5 litre conical flask and make up to 2 litres with distilled water. Mix until dissolved and plug the flask with cotton wool. Filter, under suction, through two sheets of Whatman No. 42 filter paper and autoclave the filtrate at 2 bar for 10 minutes. Allow to cool to room temperature before use.

4. Two units of concentrated human red cells, either fresh or time expired but certainly donated less than 30 days previously, should be obtained by arrangement with the Blood Transfusion Service. Each unit of red cells is filtered under gravity through the standard filter of a clinical blood giving set into an evacuated 400 ml transfer pack.

5. For each pack of red cells prepare a mixture of 250 ml of the Alsever's solution to which has been added 0.8 ml of a 50 per cent aqueous solution of glutaraldehyde. Mix well and add to the red cells noting the time at which the first drops of this solution come into contact with the red cells. The suspension of cells in gluteraldehyde is mixed for 30 seconds and left at room temperature for a total of five minutes from the time of addition of the glutaraldehyde. After this time spin down the red cells at 1800 g for 10 minutes at a temperature of 4°C. Remove the supernatant and top layer of cells immediately after centrifugation. It is important that the total time between the addition of the first drops of glutaraldehyde and the removal of the glutaraldehyde-containing supernatant should not exceed 25 min. The cells are then resuspended in 200 ml of Alsever's solution (without glutaraldehyde), centrifuged and the supernatant and top layer of cells removed. This washing process is carried out four times to remove all traces of the glutaraldehyde.

6. Estimate the volume of concentrated red cells and their hemoglobin concentration and calculate the amount of Alsever's solution to be added to the cells to give a final Hb concentration of about 13 g/dl. Do not add this solution yet.

Preparation of the whole blood control

7. Calculate the total volume of the cells and Alsever's solution together. Add to the Alsever's solution the appropriate quantities of disodium ethylene diamine tetraacetic acid (EDTA), chloromycetin succinate and neomycin sulphate to give concentrations in the mixed cells and Alsever's solution of 20g/l EDTA, 500 mg/l chloromycetin succinate and 170 mg/l neomycin sulphate. Add these compounds to the required amount of Alsever's solution and, when fully dis-

solved, filter the solution through two layers of Whatman No. 42 filter paper under suction. Add this solution to the red cells and mix thoroughly.

8. Estimate the nucleated (white) cell count of the mixture using a Coulter S. Wait for two minutes and recount the same sample using the 'count' button on the control panel. The nucleated cell count should be constant and less than $2 \times 10^9/l$. Pour the reconstituted blood into a sterile Winchester bottle and mix for 10 min.

9. The fixed chicken red cells, to be used as a white cell analogue, should be mixed thoroughly for 20 min. Calculate the amount required to give a nucleated cell count of about $8 \times 10^9/l$ when added to the stabilized human red cells. Slowly add this amount to the human red cell suspension, mixing thoroughly all the while. After addition of the fixed chicken red cells allow the contents of the Winchester bottle to mix for a further 30 min then remove two 20 ml aliquots and place them in plastic screw-topped universal containers. Store the reconstituted blood in the Winchester and the two aliquots at 4°C.

10. This reconstituted blood takes approximately three to four weeks to achieve complete stability. During this period the aliquots should be assayed on the Coulter S about once every three days. The mean cell volume (MCV) takes the longest time to stabilize. The reconstituted whole blood is ready for use as a control when two values of the MCV obtained at least three days apart are the same.

11. When the blood has fully stabilized it should be dispensed into 15–20 ml aliquots as necessary to allow convenient use in the laboratory. This is best achieved using the type of continuous mixing and dispensing device described by Ward et al.[15] Check for homogeneity of dispensing between bottles by taking a one in fifty random selection. Variation of results between bottles should not be greater than that from within the bottles.

Procedure for handling the whole blood control
The cells in the whole blood control tend to become 'sticky' and to agglutinate. They must be thoroughly mixed before use. A suitable procedure is described below. The blood should be stored at 4 to 10°C.

Use only one bottle at a time and remove it from storage at least 45 min before use. During this time it should be gently but continuously mixed on a rocker-roller mixer. The blood should not be shaken, nor should glass beads be added to facilitate mixing. Before use ensure that no cells still adhere to the container wall. Continue to mix until this occurs.

The blood should be left to stand upright for 20 s before sampling to allow any bubbles to escape to the surface. After the initial mixing period the blood may be left to stand for most of the time but requires 2 min mixing before sampling.

This blood is specifically prepared for use with the Coulter S. It may not be suitable for use with other automated blood counters.

B. CALIBRATING THE COULTER S

There is no generally accepted whole blood standard for hematology. Methods of standardizing blood counters are described in Chapter 2.

C. ESTABLISHING THE MEAN AND VARIANCE OF THE CONTROL BLOOD IN THE TEST PROCEDURE, AND THE QUALITY CONTROL LIMITS

The mean (and variance) of the control blood is established each time a batch of the blood is ready for use. These values are determined from a minimum of ten replicate measurements.

1. Ensure that the blood counter is properly standardized.
2. Analyze ten or more replicate samples of the control blood from one 20 ml aliquot. Precede each control sample by a sample of ISOTON to ensure that the carry-over is the same for each sample. Calculate the mean of the results of the control blood samples and their variance (see Appendix).
3. The parameters of the quality control scheme should now be calculated. The decision interval scheme is the most appropriate and simple to use for a busy laboratory. Quality control of all the parameters determined by the Coulter S is not necessary. The four directly measured parameters, the white blood cell count (WBC), red blood cell count (RBC), hemoglobin concentration (Hb) and mean corpuscular volume (MCV) should be subject to quality control. Calculate the upper reference value (URV) and lower reference value (LRV) for each of these parameters from the formulae:

URVs Wbc = mean + 0.3
      Rbc = mean + 0.05
      Hb = mean + 0.1
      MCV = mean + 1
LRVs Wbc = mean − 0.3
      Rbc = mean − 0.05
      Hb = mean − 0.1
      MCV = mean − 1

Set decision intervals as follows
      Wbc = ± 0.7
      Rbc = ± 0.13
      Hb = ± 0.3
      MCV = ± 3

The positive values are used as the upper decision intervals (UDI) and the negative values are used as the lower decision intervals (LDI).

Sometimes the mean for one of the parameters falls between two of the values which the Coulter S can print. For example, the mean haemoglobin concentration might be 13.25 although the Coulter S provides results of only 13.2 or 13.3 g/dl. Under such circumstances it is useful to take the nearest number above the mean (e.g. 13.3) as the mean for calculating the URV and the nearest number below (e.g. 13.2) as the mean for calculating the LRV. As a rule of thumb, if the mean of any parameter is in the middle of the range between two possible result values, that is between 0.25 and 0.75 of the last significant digit, then round up to calculate the URV and round down to calculate the LRV. Otherwise round to the nearest possible result and use the same value for both the URV and LRV. The decision intervals are unaffected by this process.

D. ANALYZING CONTROL SAMPLES IN THE WORKFLOW

A control sample should be tested after approximately every 20 cycles of the Coulter S. Under some circumstances, such as when a malfunction is suspected, it is advisable to analyze control samples more frequently. Each control sample should be preceded by a sample of ISOTON to eliminate any effect of carry-over. No further patients' samples should be analyzed until the analysis of the control results has been completed and any corrective action, such as recalibration, has been undertaken if necessary.

E. ANALYSIS OF THE QUALITY CONTROL RESULTS AND TESTING FOR CHANGES

Record the values of the control parameters on a worksheet such as that shown in Figure 8.2. Then, starting with a cusum of zero:
1. If the control value lies between the two reference values do not start a cusum.
2. If the control value falls outside the reference values start a cusum of the difference between the result and the appropriate reference value.
3. Continue calculating the cusum on subsequent control results using the same reference value. The cusum should be calculated even when the result lies between the two reference values, or even outside the opposite reference value.
4. If, during a cusum calculation, the cusum returns to zero or changes sign, set the cusum to zero.
5. If a cusum changes sign because the control result lies outside the opposite reference value, check the test procedure as in B below. This should be taken as an indication of a possible abrupt change in calibration.
6. If the cusum equals or exceeds the decision interval a significant change in accuracy has probably occurred. Set the cusum to zero. Check the performance of the test procedure as described below.

   Two types of change in accuracy may occur. A small but consistent change is the more common and it is this that the cusum technique is ideally suited to detect. It is characterized by a small but steady rise in the magnitude of the cusum until it reaches the decision interval. Occasionally, however, a control result may deviate markedly from the mean value such that in one sample the cusum may leap from zero to a level exceeding the decision interval or from a positive to a large negative value (or vice versa). It is not always obvious whether this represents a real large change in accuracy or is simply the result of one of the sporadic and inexplicable rogue results which bedevil laboratory life. It is therefore useful to evaluate these two types of change in different ways.

   A. Small but consistent changes are a real indication of a loss of accuracy and the calibration of the machine should be checked.

   B. When it is suspected that there has been a large sudden change, such as a change in sign of a cusum, or a rogue result, the performance of the test procedure should be checked using the control blood. Analyze three control samples,

preceding each by a sample of ISOTON. Assess the accuracy by the standard cusum technique starting with the cusum at zero. If the cusum does not exceed the decision interval for any of the three samples resume the analysis of patients' samples and controls: it was probably a single rogue result. If the cusum exceeds the decision interval for any of the samples then check the calibration as described in A above.

F. CORRECTIVE AND SUBSEQUENT ACTION

The appropriate way of detecting faults is fully described in the instruction manual for the Coulter S and amplified in Chapter 2. Always check the obvious, such as a blocked sample valve or loss of diluent, first. When a fault has been identified and corrected the calibration of the machine should be checked as in A above. In most cases there will be no need to recalibrate; once the fault is remedied the analyzer will be correctly calibrated. In some cases recalibration will also be required.

When no cause of the change can be determined yet the analyzer needs to be recalibrated there may remain the suspicion that all is not well. In these circumstances it is useful to analyze control samples more frequently than usual. A practical approach is to analyze the following three control samples after every ten cycles of the analyzer, rather than after every 20 cycles. If there is no evidence of any change after the first three samples have been analyzed then the control sampling regime can revert to normal. If a fault continues then an increased frequency of sampling will allow it to be detected more rapidly than usual.

MODIFICATIONS TO THE CONTROL SCHEME TO ALLOW MONITORING OF PRECISION

The method of quality control described above is aimed at control of the accuracy of a test procedure by analyzing a single sample of a control blood at regular intervals. If it is necessary to assess changes in precision then the technique must be modified to allow duplicate estimation of the control blood values on each occasion. For most practical purposes, duplicate results are sufficient to provide an adequate degree of control. Assaying the control blood in triplicate or more is impracticable in the face of the workload of most laboratories. The use of duplicates requires changes in the control scheme for accuracy, as well as allowing control of precision.

Accuracy

The cusum calculations are based on the mean value of the two observations. Accordingly, all calculations, including the setting of reference values and decision intervals, should be carried out to the nearest 0.5 of the least significant unit of each result printed by the Coulter S. That is, all figures should be rounded to the nearest 0.05 for the Wbc, 0.005 for the Rbc, 0.05 for the Hb and 0.5 for the MCV. In addition, the reference values and decision intervals must be multiplied by a factor of $1/\sqrt{2}$ to allow for duplicates. For this scheme the reference values should be set at the following distance from the mean:

Wbc   ± 0.20
Rbc   ± 0.035
Hb   ± 0.05
MCV   ± 0.5

The decision intervals for the new scheme are:
Wbc   ± 0.45
Rbc   ± 0.090
Hb   ± 0.20
MCV   ± 2.0

All other aspects of the control scheme for accuracy are unaltered.

Precision

The sample variance of each pair of duplicate measurements on the control blood is calculated from the formula:

$$s^2 = \tfrac{1}{2}(x_1 - x_2)^2$$

where the duplicate results are x_1 and x_2. This is divided by the variance of the test procedure to give an index, C, of the variability of the procedure at that point: $C = s^2/\sigma^2$. Suitable estimates of the variance, σ^2, for each of the four parameters measured by the Coulter S are:

Wbc   0.06
Rbc   0.0025
Hb   0.01
MCV   1

The difference between this ratio, C, and its target value, 1, is then calculated for each pair of data: diff = C − 1. The cusum of these differences for each successive pair of data is then calculated simply by adding each to the preceding sum. This precision cusum can then be plotted in exactly the same manner as the cusum for monitoring accuracy.

A suitable decision interval scheme can also be used to monitor precision in a similar way to that by which accuracy was monitored and using the same worksheet as that shown in Figure 8.2. In this case the 'Result' is in the index of precision: $\tfrac{1}{2} \cdot \dfrac{(x_1 - x_2)^2}{\sigma^2}$. The 'Cusum' is calculated about the upper or lower reference values in the usual way. Because the control statistics for all parameters are expressed in terms of the variance of the test procedure for that parameter the target mean, decision intervals and reference values are the same for all. These values are calculated from d and tan θ given in Table 8.1. For duplicate determinations the appropriate formula is:

$$k = 2\sqrt{2}\tan\theta = 0.84$$
$$h = 2\sqrt{2}\,d\tan\theta = 8.50$$

Thus reference values are set at 1 ± k where k = 0.84, that is 0.16 and 1.84 for the LRV and URV respectively. The decision interval is always h = ± 8.50. This scheme will detect a change in precision of the test procedure by a factor of 2 within, on average, 6 control samples of the change occurring and will give false positive indications no more than once in every 300 control evaluations.

When control samples are assayed in triplicate at each point then the characteristics of the decision interval scheme derived from the V-mask (Table 8.1) are given by:

$$k = 2 \tan \theta$$
$$h = 2 d \tan \theta$$

Thus, for example, if control samples are analysed in triplicate the sample variance is calculated as using the standard statistical formula (see Appendix — Simple Statistics), and the control statistic is still $C = s^2/\sigma^2$. Suitable reference values and decision intervals in this case would be:

$$k = \pm 0.84$$
$$h = \pm 5.40$$

This scheme would detect changes in precision by a factor of 2 within 4 control evaluations of the change occurring and potentially give false positive warnings only once in every 560 control samples.

The cusum calculations and methods of evaluation proceed exactly as for the control of accuracy. Evaluating the cause and significance of the change is more difficult. A suggested procedure would be as follows:

1. Make 10 replicate measurements of the control blood, preceding each by a sample of ISOTON as usual.
2. Calculate the variance of these results and divide this by the variance of the test procedure to give a variance ratio, F.
3. If F is between 1.84 and 0.54 assume that no real change has occurred. These are the minimum changes which the quality control scheme can detect.
4. If F is greater than 1.84 or less than 0.54 then a change of precision has occurred.

When a change in precision, usually an increase rather than a decrease in variance, has occurred than this is a firm indication that the estimation has become erratic. A change in accuracy may occur simultaneously. The machine should be thoroughly checked any malfunction rectified and recalibrated appropriately.

AUTOMATION OF QUALITY CONTROL

Providing and practising an adequate system of quality control in a hematology laboratory is not to be undertaken lightly. It is a moderately expensive process, both in terms of materials and, particularly, time. Nevertheless, quality control should be an integral part of laboratory practice. Throughout this chapter the emphasis has been on the detection of faults in a test procedure. This is a rather negative attitude. The primary function of a quality control system is to give a positive indication that the test procedure is functioning satisfactorily. The time and resources involved in running such a system may have discouraged many overworked laboratories from providing good quality control. Automation of the simple arithmetical processes for analyzing control results is invaluable in a busy laboratory. The advent of a variety of powerful calculators and the increasing use of computers in hematology laboratories can produce a considerable saving in the time and effort involved in quality control. When the calculations are carried out automatically the problems of maintaining quality control become trivial. About three-quarters of the time involved is taken up by the calculations: this may take up to one-and-a-half hours of technician time each day for the Coulter S. The use of a computer can reduce this to a few seconds and it has been suggested[16] that this may be one of the more relevant applications of computers in hematology.

The principle of quality control for all parameters is the same; the only things which vary are the test statistics, which are different for the control of accuracy and precision, and the reference values and decision intervals. These are different for each parameter for the control of accuracy but identical for all parameters for the control of precision provided the same properties of the control scheme are required for each. The arithmetic calculations are identical for analyzing any cusum chart.

A simple flow diagram for the calculations and decisions made from them has been described by Cavill and Ricketts.[2] Because a continuous list of the control results and cusums may not be available to the operator when a computer is used, they may be stored internally, this flow chart may need to be modified to provide specific warning of sudden large changes and to assess changes in precision.

A variety of equipment can be used to perform the calculations but whatever is used the calculations must be performed immediately, before proceeding with the analysis of further patients' blood samples. By this means the laboratory can be positively confident about the results that is produces and can say that if a result has been issued then it was the product of a method that was in control: whether the sample was satisfactory is another matter. For maximum efficiency the Coulter S, or any other automated blood analysis equipment, should be directly linked to the computer. An off-line system in which the results are processed in batches at infrequent intervals, for example daily, can not be used to provide real-time quality control.

A programmable calculator can be used to perform the necessary calculations. For this to be worthwhile the calculator must have certain characteristics. It must be able to store the cusums for each parameter for the lifetime of a control preparation which will usually be one month; it must also be capable of storing the reference values and the decision intervals. In addition, there must be sufficient program steps available to complete the calculations and, most important, the calculator must be able to test whether a number is greater than zero and branch the program accordingly.

OTHER HEMATOLOGICAL TESTS

This chapter has been concerned with quality control of automated blood counters, particularly the Coulter S and its relatives. This is because routine blood counts probably account for about two-thirds of the numerical results produced by a hematology laboratory and because it is the most highly automated of laboratory procedures. The use of control samples and cumulative sum techniques is not, however, limited to blood counting. They can be, and are, used for monitoring the performance of a variety of hematological tests which produce numerical, rather than qualitative, results. As other techniques become more automated and the demand for them increases so must the application of active quality control become more widespread.

The control preparation needs to be stable over a long period. For quality control of many serum or plasma constituents human serum derived from therapeutic phlebotomies and stored in aliquots at $-20°C$ is suitable. This has been used in this laboratory for quality control of serum vitamin B_{12}, folate, ferritin and, when the assay is still occassionally carried out, serum iron concentrations. The control samples are inserted in the batches after approximately every 20 patients' samples. A minimum of four quality control samples are included in any one batch of assays. The fact that the test is performed as a batch does not change the quality control method. The results of the control samples should still be the same from batch to batch. The only slight modification that needs to be made to this approach is in evaluating the results. This arises because the results are often not known until all the samples have been analyzed and then they all become available simultaneously. Nevertheless they should be analyzed in the appropriate order. If there is no evidence of any change the results for the complete batch can be issued. When, on the other hand, one of the control results indicates a change then only the patients' samples analyzed before control may be assumed to be correct. In most cases it will be worthwhile examining the subsequent control results to determine whether the change has been sustained for the rest of the batch. There are no hard and fast rules for assessing this. A suitable rule of thumb is:

1. If there are four or more additional control samples, reset the cusum to zero and start a new cusum for the additional samples. If this indicates a loss of control, then the change has been sustained and the patients' samples need to be reassayed. If no further loss of control is indicated then reassay the patients' samples between the control sample which indicated a change and the subsequent one. All other patients' samples should be correct.
2. If there are three or less additional control samples calculate their mean value. If this falls outside the reference values assume that the change has been sustained. Otherwise the change was probably transient. In each case, treat the patients' samples as in (i) above.

The usefulness of control samples and cusum techniques for monitoring hematological tests other than routine blood counting cannot be overemphasized.

CONCLUSIONS

Two recent developments will allow the introduction of a sensitive and comprehensive system of quality control to a wide variety of test procedures in haematology. The main limitation to quality control of routine blood counting has been the provision of a stable whole blood to use as a control preparation. The development described by Morgan et al[1] has removed this constraint and allowed quality control of blood counting to be placed on a firm basis. The second development[14] of formulae for cusum schemes for the control of precision means that both the accuracy and the precision of a test procedure can be continuously assessed. Monitoring accuracy and monitoring precision are not alternative procedures: they are complementary.

Control samples and cumulative sum techniques provide a sensitive and effective method of quality control. They are simple to use and can easily be automated. Quality control of a variety of hematological test procedures is essential and the methods described in this chapter provide a practical approach to the problems involved.

REFERENCES

1. Morgan L O, Jones W G, Fisher J, Cavill I 1978 A whole blood control for the Coulter Model S. Journal of Clinical Pathology 31: 50–53
2. Cavill I, Ricketts C 1974 Automated quality control for the haematology laboratory. Journal of Clinical Pathology 27: 757–759
3. Cavill I 1971 Quality control in routine haemoglobinometry. Journal of Clinical Pathology 24: 701–704
4. Cavill I, Jacobs A 1973 Quality control in haematology. Association of Clinical Pathologists, Broadsheet 75
5. Whole blood standards for use in haematology. GB Patent Specification 1509539. 4th May 1978
6. International Committee for Standardization in Haematology 1967 Recommendations for haemoglobinometry in human blood. British Journal of Haematology 13 supplement: 71–75
7. International Committee for Standardization in Haematology 1971 Proposed recommendations for the measurement of serum iron in human blood. British Journal of Haematology 20: 451–453
8. Barnard G A 1959 Control charts and stochastic processes. Journal of the Royal Statistical Society, Series B 21: 239–271
9. Wetherill G B 1969 Sampling inspection and quality control. Methuen, London
10. Ewan W D, Kemp K W 1960 Sampling inspection of continuous processes with no autocorrelation between successive results. Biometrika 47: 363–380
11. Goldsmith P L, Whitfield H 1961 Average run lengths in cumulative chart quality control schemes. Technometrics 3: 11–20
12. Wilson D W, Griffiths K, Kemp K W, Nix A B J, Rowlands R J 1979 Internal quality control of radioimmunoassays: monitoring of error. Journal of Endocrinology 80: 365–372
13. Pearson E S, Hartley H O 1966 Biometrika Tables for Statisticians, 3rd edn. Cambridge, Cambridge University Press

14. Rowlands R J 1976 Formulae for performance characteristics of cumulative schemes when observations are autocorrelated. PhD thesis, University of Wales
15. Ward P G, Chappell D A, Fox J G C 1975 Mixing and bottling unit for preparing biological fluids used in quality control. Laboratory Practice 24: 577–583
16. Cavill I, Ricketts C, Jacobs A 1975 Computers in Haematology. Butterworth, London.

9
The Interpretation and Significance of Laboratory Results
I. Cavill   A. Jacobs

The clinical hematology laboratory aims to provide, as one of its main functions, quantitative data on physiological and biochemical characteristics of blood which have a bearing on the care and management of patients. These patients generally have but one objective in mind — that is to solve their major medical problems as quickly as possible. Laboratory investigations are ultimately justified only by their effectiveness in helping to gain this objective. Quality control can make a significant contribution towards this by ensuring that any results issued by the laboratory give a true measure of the parameter concerned. Even the most accurate result will be worthless if the clinician managing the patient does not have confidence in the data and an understanding of its limitations. In this respect it is important of distinguish between the accuracy and precision of a measurement and the variability of that parameter in human subjects. For example, it is possible to measure serum iron concentration with great accuracy, yet a variation in the iron concentration of 100 per cent or more between successive samples in the same patient may have no pathological significance. In vivo, the serum iron concentration is extremely labile and may vary in the same person during a single day between 'normal' or even 'high' levels down to a concentration which is commonly associated with iron deficiency. In this brief chapter we shall therefore try to add a clinical perspective to the pursuit of accuracy and precision within the laboratory.

The first problem in defining variation in vivo is to ensure methodological constancy. The particular difficulty in hematology, as has already been stressed in previous chapters, is the absence of standard materials, particularly in blood counting. In part this is overcome by using indirect methods of calibration and control in which artificial preparations imitating whole blood are used. Such preparations will differ in many respects from fresh blood samples and it has been argued that the use of preserved control preparations may not reflect methodological changes which would affect fresh clinical samples. The possibility of age related changes within control preparations leading to a false indication of loss of accuracy or giving rise to erroneous changes in calibration has also limited their use in some laboratories. It has long been suggested that the ideal control material for blood counting would be samples taken from the same reference individual at appropriate times and analyzed as fresh blood. Because the daily turnover of red cells is of the order of 1 per cent the cells present in the circulation on any one day will be much the same as those on the next day in a normal subject in a physiologically stable state. Although the concentration of cells, reflected in the red cell count (RBC) hemoglobin concentration (Hb) and packed cell volume (PCV) may change from sample to sample the characteristics of the individual cells (mean corpuscular volume (MCV), mean corpuscular hemoglobin (MCH), and mean corpuscular hemoglobin concentration (MCHC)) should not vary from day to day.

In order to try and explore this problem we recently studied a group of normal subjects. Venous blood samples were taken at regular intervals over a two-month period. At the same time that the fresh blood samples were analyzed in triplicate a sample of Coulter 4C Control material was also measured ten times. The Coulter Model S blood counter used for these measurements was calibrated so that the MCV, MCH and MCHC of the subjects remained constant throughout the study. As can be seen from Figure 9.1, the red cell indices for the 4C material remained steady throughout two months' observation. This led us to conclude that as far as these indices were concerned we could continue to use either Coulter 4C, or a material which have been shown to be as stable, for the long term control of these parameters. Furthermore, as the hemoglobin concentration of the 4C Control remained stable during this time we could be confident that the red cell counts were also stable. There was therefore no reason to suppose that there had been any deterioration in the material over the two months of the study, and rather than attack the veins of a band of volunteers to maintain constancy it would be equally acceptable to use the Coulter 4C material itself.

During this study the results from patient samples which were measured at the same time as the blood from the control subjects were analyzed by the method described by Korpman and Bull.[1] When data from patients attending hematology outpatients clinics were excluded then variation in the running

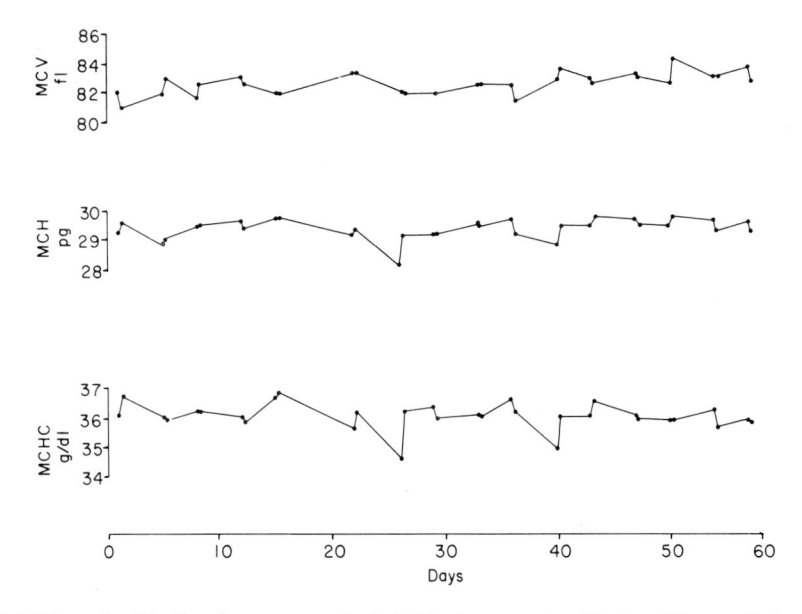

Fig. 9.1 The red cell indices for a preserved whole blood preparation (Coulter 4C) over 60 days.

mean of the red cell indices was generally less than 3 per cent. There were a number of occasions when the mean deviated by more than 2 per cent from the population mean. This probably resulted from the non-random arrival of samples in the laboratory from particular groups of patients and from changes in the population of patients from day to day. This problem and a method for stabilizing the data are described in Chapter 5. In some circumstances however the very stability of the moving average may obscure real changes in machine calibration[2] (Fig. 9.2). This approach cannot be applied to parameters where the distribution of patients results may vary from day to day and week to week as is the case, for example, with hemoglobin concentration and white cell count.[3] Nevertheless, when the characteristics of the incoming patient samples are sufficiently constant and the sequence of analysis of samples is sufficiently randomized (Ch. 5) then it is clearly possible to use patients' data as the control material for the red cell indices. These caveats do not apply to the use of preserved control materials provided that the characteristics of such materials have proved to be stable. Unlike patients samples, which are in abundant supply and

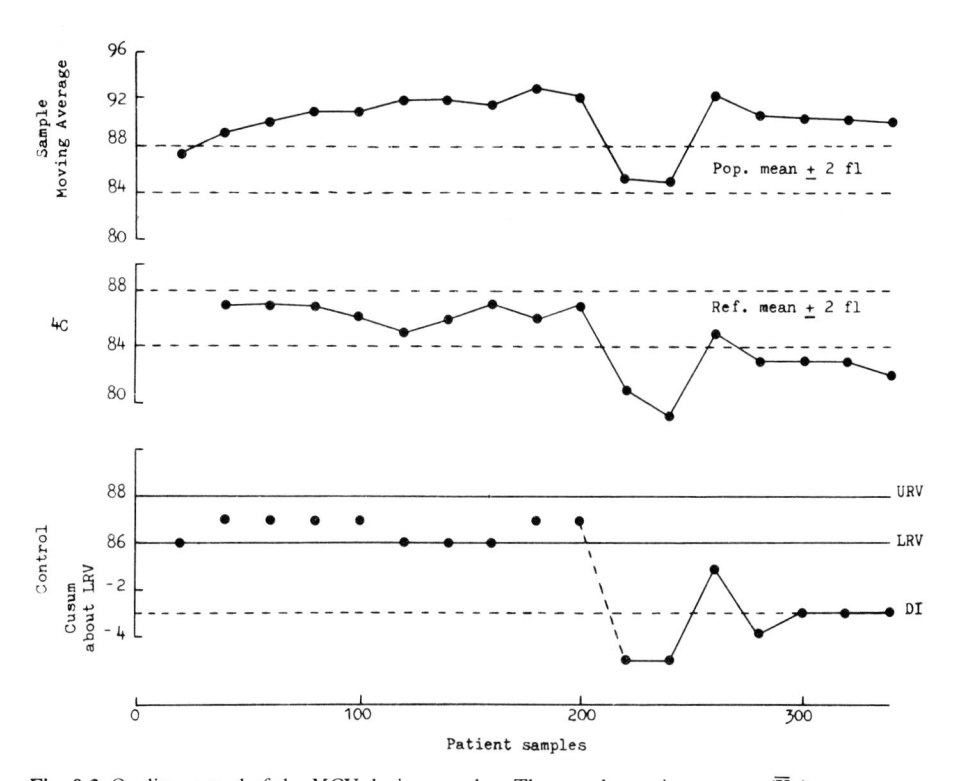

Fig. 9.2 Quality control of the MCV during one day. The sample moving average ($\overline{X}_B$) was calculated after every 20 patient samples. At the same time a sample of Coulter 4C and another preserved blood control were also analyzed. The acceptable limits for $\overline{X}_B$ and the Coulter 4C are indicated by dashed lines. The results from the control blood are plotted between the upper and lower reference values (URV and LRV): the points below the LRV represent a cusum whose decision interval (DI) is indicated by a dashed line.

A mis-calibration was introduced after the 200th patient sample. (From Cavill et al 1979.[2])

involve no extra cost in time or money, stable control materials must either be purchased or specially prepared.

Having established methodological constancy it is then possible to make some estimate of the degree of variability of hematological parameters in a given subject. The laboratory should be able to give the clinician an indication of when a difference between two sequential results is pathologically significant. This is unrelated to the concept of a normal range but concentrates on detecting hematological change in a single individual. In the case of the hemoglobin concentration variations in blood sampling techniques between different phlebotomists are known to produce small but sometimes significant changes in hemoglobin concentrations of the blood samples. Despite this, the evidence[4] indicates that in the absence of disease the hemoglobin concentration in a single individual is remarkably constant. The maximum day-to-day coefficient of variation of this parameter is less than 3 per cent. At a hemoglobin concentration of 14.8 g/dl this means that two successive measurements should be within 0.4 g/dl of the mean and that the difference between such measurements should be less than 0.9 g/dl. Variations less than that should not necessarily be attributed to pathological change. However, it is still possible for smaller changes to be pathologically significant if a succession of samples show a consistent trend. The difficulty in detecting such changes in patient samples is exactly the same as that described earlier for quality control samples and application of the same cusum method (Ch. 1) is equally valid if a critical analysis is required.

As far as cell counts are concerned the red cells appear to be as stable as the hemoglobin concentrations and the day to day coefficient of variation is less than 3 per cent.[4,5] Thus at a red cell count of $500 \times 10^9/l$ no two counts should differ by more than $0.30 \times 10^{12}/l$ unless the balance of red cell production and destruction is disturbed. However, the coefficient of variation for the total leukocyte count in whole blood may be between 12 and 16 per cent[4] even when carried out by accurate automated apparatus. This means that for leukocyte counts in the region of $7.0 \times 10^9/l$ the count for any individual may very well vary by $2.2 \times 10^9/l$ between successive counts as a result of chance alone. Although exercise has been said to increase the white cell count a systematic study provided no evidence of any significant relationship between activity prior to blood sampling and the measured total white cell count.[5]

The stability of the 'absolute' red cell indices is a hematological axiom. However, a recent observation that the MCV measured by the Coulter S Counter was raised in patients with hyperosomolar plasma has suggested that the red cell cell volume may not be constant. When red cells becomes loaded with d-glucose as a result of intravenous infusions this does not equilibrate rapidly with the extracellular fluid. As a result when the blood is diluted within the automatic counter the cells will be effectively hypertonic with respect to the diluent and will swell accordingly.[6] Although this appears to be an in vitro phenomenon the possibility that in vivo changes in the plasma may also have an effect on the MCV cannot be ignored. The lesson of this observation is that no measurement is 'absolute' and that the hematologist must be constantly aware of the possibility of unexpected factors influencing the data emerging from even the best 'controlled' laboratory.

The variability of the platelet count which might be expected in a normal subject is entirely related to the method of counting. The clinician is often unaware of this and may have no knowledge of the method used on his behalf. Modern automated apparatus is quite capable of measuring platelet numbers with an accuracy of 1 to 2 per cent but 'manual' methods which rely upon visual counting can be extremely inaccurate. Cell counts approximate to the Poisson distribution (Ch. 1) so that it is possible to calculate the coefficient of variation of the number of cells observed from the square root of that count. Thus for a platelet count of $120 \times 10^9/l$ where the total number of platelets seen in the counting chamber was 120 the coefficient of variation of the count would be 9 per cent. This means only that the true number of cells in the chamber could lie in the range 109 to 131 and occasionally be anywhere in the region of 100 to 140. The derived platelet count would have the same degree of inaccuracy. Even when accurate automated methods of platelet counting are used the expected day to day variation in any subject is much greater than for the red cell count because of physiological fluctuations. In normal subjects there may be a coefficient of variation of 13 per cent although the hour to hour variation is generally less than 2 per cent.[4,5] Thus in the region of a platelet count of $120 \times 10^9/l$ results on successive days might be expected to differ by up to $31 \times 10^9/l$. When the count is made by a well controlled accurate automated method it would be unwise to attribute any difference of less than $30 \times 10^9/l$ between successive counts to pathological change. For manually counted platelets it might be prudent to double that figure.

The differential leukocyte count as practised in most routine hematology laboratories suffers from an even greater degree of inaccuracy than the manual estimation of the platelet count. When the differential is based on the examination of only 100 white cells the accuracy of the neutrophil count will be in the region of ±14 per cent while that for the less frequent cell types, such as eosinophils, may be in the region of ±50 per cent. Using methods based on only the 100 cell differential the day-to-day coefficient of variation for neutrophils and lymphocytes are both in the region of 20 per cent.[5] Rather surprisingly, when the neutrophil count was estimated by an automated method in which the analytical variation had been reduced to 2.5 per cent the physiological variation within a single subject was found to be even greater (coefficient of variation 26 per cent)[4] than for the manual method. There appears to be no consistent pattern to this variation and it seems likely that the lability of the white cell count is related to the short intravascular lifespan and high turnover rate of the cells. In view of the methodological inaccuracies inherent in the differential count based on 100 cells it could be argued that any apparently quantitative result would be fraudulent and that a comment on the predominant cell type seen in a blood film and a note on the presence of minority populations would be as clinically useful and at least more truthful. Indeed it has been suggested[7] that the importance of the differential is simply that 'it assures the attending physician that a qualified morphologist, after having examined the peripheral blood film for approximately 90 seconds, has failed to find any significant abnormality'. There seems to be no point in automating the differential count if only 100 or 200 white cells are counted. Producing more bad results more easily does not make for better hematology. The proper use of automation in this field would seem to be to increase the accuracy of the differential white cell count. This can be done by automatic examination of a far larger number of cells. Unfortunately automated techniques based on histochemical staining of cells may result in a difference between the criteria for characterizing particular cell types and those used in classical Romanowsky staining. This needs further evaluation especially in abnormal blood samples. Even when differential counting techniques have been perfected there will still be considerable biological variability and the time has probably now come for a clinical assessment of the value of the differential count on the basis of accurate methods.

For the large number of other hematological investigations carried out routinely the normal physiological variability of the results is generally not well defined. Random samples for diagnostic purposes have therefore to be interpreted with great caution. The variability of the serum iron concentration with marked and unpredictable changes occurring during a period of a few minutes has already been described (Fig. 9.3). Similarly, serum folate concentrations vary according to the time of day and relationship to the last (possibly folate-containing) meal. In addition there may well be interaction between blood constituents which may affect the result for a particular parameter. Platelet function tests may be influenced by recent aspirin ingestion and serum ferritin concentration by ascorbic acid status.

Most hematology laboratories issue reports which are not based on simple numerical data. Qualitative results, especially of morphological or cytochemical studies, are equally worthy of quality control. Some attempts at standardization of this aspect of hematology has been attempted in a number of countries and the experience of the Laboratory Proficiency Testing Program (LPTP) in Onta-

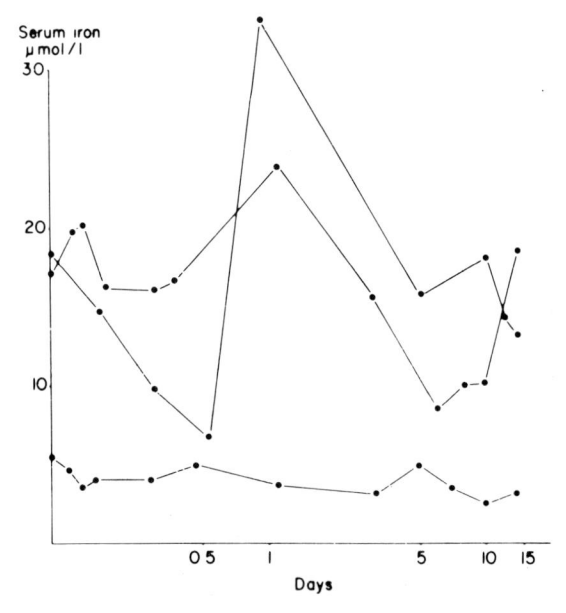

Fig. 9.3 The serum iron concentration in two norml subjects (upper lines) and an iron deficient patient over 15 days (the time scale is plotted logarithmically).

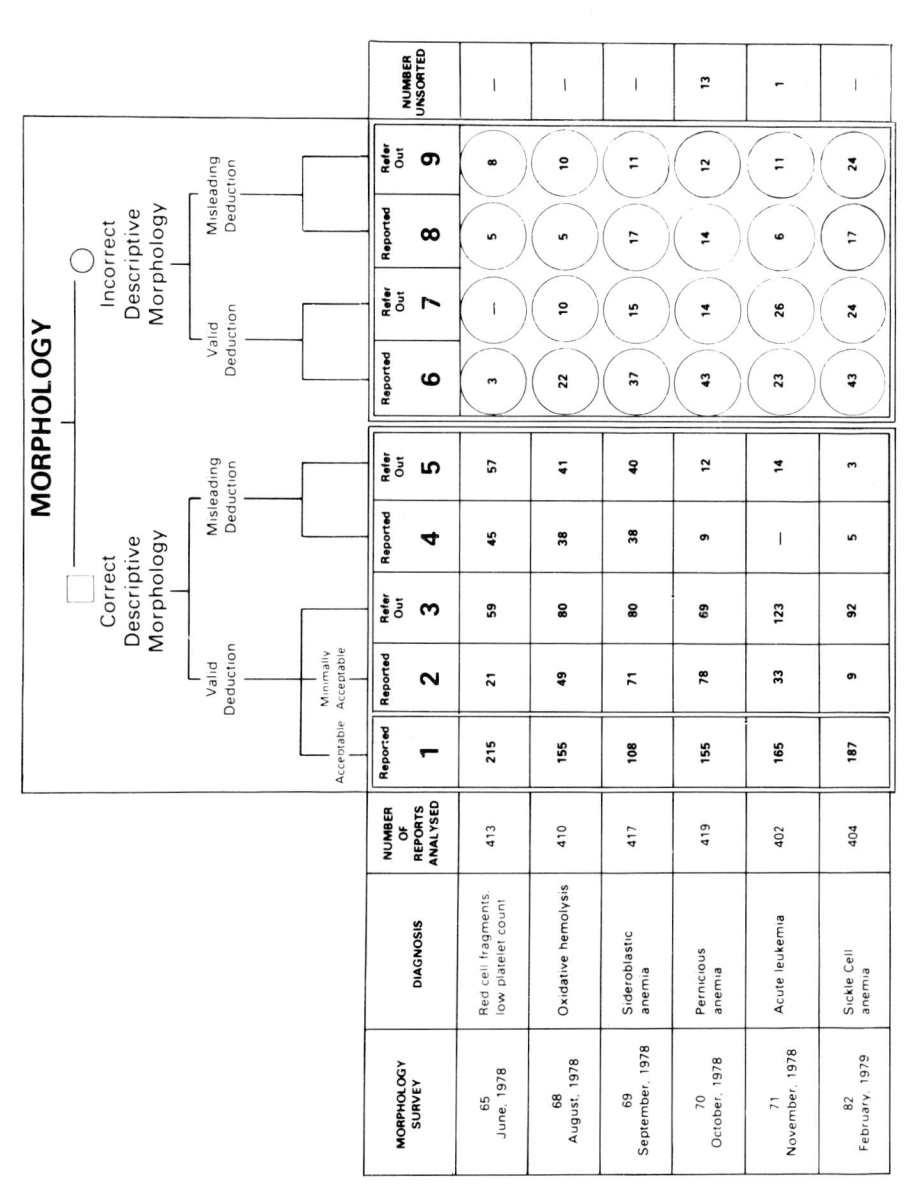

THE INTERPRETATION AND SIGNIFICANCE OF LABORATORY RESULTS 179

MORPHOLOGY SURVEY	DIAGNOSIS	NUMBER OF REPORTS ANALYSED	Reported 1	Reported 2	Refer Out 3	Reported 4	Refer Out 5	Reported 6	Refer Out 7	Reported 8	Refer Out 9	NUMBER UNSORTED
65 June, 1978	Red cell fragments low platelet count	413	215	21	59	45	57	3	—	5	8	—
68 August, 1978	Oxidative hemolysis	410	155	49	80	38	41	22	10	5	10	—
69 September, 1978	Sideroblastic anemia	417	108	71	80	38	40	37	15	17	11	—
70 October, 1978	Pernicious anemia	419	155	78	69	9	12	43	14	14	12	13
71 November, 1978	Acute leukemia	402	165	33	123	—	14	23	26	6	11	1
82 February, 1979	Sickle Cell anemia	404	187	9	92	5	3	43	24	17	24	—

Fig. 9.4 Analysis of the results from six proficiency surveys of morphological hematology in the LPTP scheme. (From Carstairs et al 1980.[8])

rio, Canada, is probably the most extensive.[8] The logistic problems associated with preparing and distributing sufficient material for several hundred widely scattered hematologists should not be underestimated. In this scheme there is no pretence that the blood films distributed are treated in the same way as the routine examinations which the laboratory carries out. The performance that is tested is therefore probably the best that can be achieved in each laboratory. This performance is judged against a yardstick of correct descriptive morphology and valid interpretation provided by a panel of 'experts'. As in all such studies the value of the exercise is related to the confidence that the participants have in the pronouncements of the 'experts'. In the LPTP scheme participants have to report on the presence of a list of characteristics, indicate what interpretation they would have made and whether or not they would have sought further expert advice. The analysis of such results (Fig. 9.4) shows that a large number of permutations are possible. Although most laboratories reported correct descriptive morphology and an acceptable interpretation there was a significant number who appeared to generate unacceptable reports. A significant minority were able to provide perfectly valid conclusions based on incorrect descriptive morphology.

The difficulties of working towards a standardized system of dealing with morphological hematology are not simply differences between laboratories. Even within one laboratory there may be divergent opinions which are partly due to differences between observers and partly due to sampling errors. For example, the study by Bentley and Williams[9] showed that when four independent observers examined 60 marrow smears stained by the Prussian-blue reaction for iron there were considerable variations in the gradings reported even though the criteria had been previously disccussed and agreed. Initial unanimous agreement was only obtained for 20 of the bone marrow smears. The disagreements were random with no evidence of consistent bias for any individual observer. In this study it was found necessary to review all the slides collectively in order to achieve a uniform and unanimous opinion. It seems likely that periodic repetition of such exercises within a laboratory might lead to mutual education and standardization.

Similar problems may arise in interpreting haematological data and arriving at a diagnosis. An initial survey in South Wales[10] provided evidence that the classification of patients suffering from leukemia could vary quite considerably between different hospitals. Complete initial agreement amongst the participants

Table 9.1 The initial grade of Perls' positive iron compared with the final agreed grade in 60 bone marrow smears. (From Bentley and Williams, 1974[9].)

Final marrow grade	Initial marrow grade			
	0	1	2	3
0	49	2	1	
1	6	16	2	
2	2	16	102	24
3			6	14

was low (56 per cent). This variability in morphological classification must be an important limitation in defining apparent differences in the incidence of a disease in different areas. Although this could also affect the subsequent management and fate of the patient the disagreements in diagnosis which would have involved the patients in a change of treatment were few (2 per cent). As a result of this study, hematologists in the area set up their own cooperative review panel. The outcome is a measure of standardization in at least this one aspect of hematology.

Our experience in the UK suggests that both hematologists and general physicians are insufficiently aware of the numerous factors affecting variability of laboratory reports, even where routine quality control procedures are in operation. Very often the clinician is unaware of the confidence limits of numerical data and the degree of observer error in subjective assessments. A critical attitude should be adopted towards all laboratory reports and especially those that do not accord with clinical observations, though clinical impressions themselves are not immune from error. Periodic review of all laboratory processes and intralaboratory discussions on methodology are both essential to the quality control process.

REFERENCES

1. Bull B S, Korpman R A 1974 The use of patient-derived hematology data in quality control. Proceedings of the San Diego Biomedical Symposium 13: 515–519
2. Cavill I, Ricketts C, Fisher J, Walpole B 1979 An evaluation of two methods of laboratory quality control. American Journal of Clinical Pathology 72: 624–627
3. Cavill I 1971 Quality control in routine haemoglobinometry. Journal of Clinical Pathology 24: 701–704
4. Statland B E, Wintel P, Harris S C, Burdsall M J, Saunders A M 1977 Evaluation of biologic sources of variation of leukocyte counts and other hematologic quantities using very precise automated analyzers. American Journal of Clinical Pathology 69: 48–54
5. Cavill I, Jacobs A, Fisher J, de Souza P 1981 Sequential blood counts and their variation in normal subjects. Clinical and Laboratory Haematology 3: 91–93
6. Allen S C, Balfour I C, Wise C C 1980 The red cell osmometer. Journal of Clinical Pathology 33: 430–433
7. Bull B S, Korpman R A 1980 Characterization of the WBC differential count. Blood Cells 6: 411–420
8. Carstairs K C, Wood D E, Jacobs W, Norman C S, Pantalong D, Poon A 1980 Morphological hematology testing under scrutiny. Ontario Medical Review 47: 167–172
9. Bentley D P, Williams, P I 1974 Serum ferritin concentration as an index of storage iron in rheumatoid arthritis. Journal of Clinical Pathology 27: 786–788
10. Whittaker J A, Withey J, Powell D E B, Parry T E, Khurshid M 1979 Leukaemia classification: a study of the accuracy of diagnosis in 456 patients. British Journal of Haematology 41: 177–184

Appendix — Simple Statistics

The statistics associated with quality control which have been mentioned throughout this volume are all related to the distribution of errors about a hypothetical true value. This means that repeated measurements of a particular parameter will give a series of results which are similar but which show differences from one another. These errors will usually have a Normal, or Gaussian, frequency distribution (see Fig. 2.2). The principle underlying the statistics derived from this distribution is that somewhere there is a true result and that the replicate measurements will tend to cluster around that true value. Although we may never know what that true result is we can get an indication of its likely whereabouts by determining what it is that the data are clustering about. There are different ways of expressing this central tendency but the most common of these averages is the mean. The mean result will not necessarily be the true result and repeated measurements of the mean will yield values which also differ one from another. The distribution of these mean results will describe the likely limits within which the true mean result may lie.

The mean ($\bar{X}$) is simply the sum of all the values divided by the number of items added (N)

$$X = \frac{\Sigma X_i}{n}$$

Although this statistic is almost intuitive it should not be underestimated. Its particular property is that it defines a value which is closer to all the results in the group than any other value. The sum of the deviations of each result from the mean (X − x) is zero. Although another point in the distribution might be closer to some results the sum of the differences between this and all the results would be greater. The mean is thus both an estimate of the underlying true result and the best representative of all the data.

The distribution of results which go to make up a particular mean can be described in a number of ways. The simplest is the range. This is, however, very easily influenced by a single aberrant result. A less readily distorted measure of the scatter of results is the sum of the squares of the differences between each value and the mean. This is the variance. The variance is, however, expressed in squared units and it is more readily comprehended as its square root, the standard deviation (SD). As has been described earlier (Ch. 1), in a Normal distribution 68.3 per cent of the results will fall within ± 1 SD about the mean. It thus describes where the bulk of the results lie and excludes aberrations and results which occur only infrequently. The size of the standard deviation will of course be related to the magnitude of the mean value. In the laboratory it is often useful to be able to compare the variability of a set of results at different levels and in order to make the standard deviation comparable at each of these levels it may be expressed as a percentage of the mean. This is more commonly known as the coefficient of variation.

The standard deviation (SD) for n observations of a parameter with values given by X_i is:

$$SD = \sqrt{\frac{\Sigma (X_i - \bar{X})^2}{n - 1}}$$

Calculating the SD using this formula has the disadvantage that the deviation from the mean $(X_i - \bar{X})$ has first to be calculated for each result. In the pre-calculator age the sum of squares of the deviations (x^2) was calculated directly from the raw data (X_i) thus:

(i) $\Sigma x^2 = \Sigma X_i^2 - \dfrac{(\Sigma X_i)^2}{n}$

(ii) Variance (Var) $= \dfrac{\Sigma x^2}{(n - 1)}$

(iii) $SD = \sqrt{\dfrac{\Sigma x^2}{n - 1}}$

From this the co-efficient of variation (CV) is given by:

$$CV = \frac{SD}{\bar{X}} \times 100\%$$

The number of samples that need to be measured in order to obtain a reasonable estimate both of the underlying true value and the variability of results about that value cannot be exactly defined. In one sense the more observations that are taken the better will be the estimate. However the return becomes disproportionately smaller as the number is increased. Although the mean will get increasingly close to the true value in proportion to the number of replicates measured the standard deviation will only decrease in proportion to the square root of that number. Thus increasing the number of replicates from 10 to 20 will only reduce the standard deviation by one-third. In practice a sample of 10 results should suffice to enable a good estimate of the mean to be obtained and to include a representative selection of results which should occur by chance alone.

The most common statistical problem that a laboratory may have to tackle is to assess whether or not one group of results differs from another. The two aspects of the mean and variability should be tackled separately. If the results are derived from replicate analyses then there is a very good chance they will have a Normal distribution and that the variances in each group will be similar. If this is so, Students t-test is appropriate. This compares the difference between two estimates of the mean with the pooled variance of the observations. If this difference is greater than could be attributed to random variation then 't' will be appropriately large.

There are two basic approaches to calculating 't' and the most common is to press the appropriate button on a pre-programmed calculator or microprocessor. The alternative is to calculate

$$t = \frac{\bar{X}_1 - \bar{X}_2}{\sqrt{\frac{Var_1}{n} + \frac{Var_2}{n}}}$$

The probability that any value of 't' may be the result of chance should be determined from 't' tables given in most statistical handbooks. The appropriate degrees of freedom under which 't' should be inspected are the total number of observations in the two groups minus two $[(n_1 + n_2) - 2]$. If this probability is less than 1 in 20 (i.e. 20:1 against or $p < 0.05$) then the difference is often felt to be significant.

The comparison of variability between two groups of data can be relatively simple. The biggest variance is divided by the smallest:

$$\frac{Var_{max}}{Var_{min}} = F$$

This F ratio gives a value whose significance can be assessed by reference to tables of 'F' values. The appropriate degrees of freedom are the number of items in each group minus one ($n_1 - 1$, $n_2 - 1$; where n_1 is the group with the greatest variance).

The laboratory may also need to assess the linearity of response of an apparatus or to compare results obtained by two different methods in a series of samples. Linear regression analysis and correlation may be a useful for either of these. In assessing linearity a sample is diluted accurately to cover the likely range of results which the method is to measure. The calculated content of each dilution is then compared with the measured result. The choice of the starting point for calculating the content of each dilution is extremely important. It is not always valid to assume that the initial undiluted sample will give the most accurate result. Choosing such a point will mask any deviation which might occur at higher levels as a result of, for example, coincidence in cell counting or deviation from linearity in spectrophotometers and radioimmunoassays. It is important to take the lowest possible value that can be accurately measured and to calculate upwards from this point if linearity of response is to be properly tested.

In comparing two methods it is obviously important to minimize any differences that might arise as a result of handling samples in a different manner for the two different methods. It is, moreover, advisable to collect a large body of data (in excess of 50 pairs) over at least several days to help minimize any problems which might be related to the particular moment rather than the method.

Least squares linear regression will not by itself indicate whether or not a series of paired data are linearly related one to another. It will simply fit the best possible straight line through the data points. Inspection of this line plotted against the data is generally sufficient to show whether or not all the points are randomly scattered about the line. If the two sets of data are similar then the slope of the line will be close to unity. The size of the slope indicates the average extent to which one method over or underestimates the other. Thus a slope of 0.8 indicates that the 'y' method gives only 80 per cent of the 'x' method; conversely a slope of 1.2 would indicate that the 'y' values were 20 per cent higher than the 'x' values. In addition, if there is no consistent displacement of one method the line will pass through the origin of the x and y axes. Thus, for a line of the form y = mx + c, m will equal 1 and c will equal 0.

The pre-calculator method of estimating the slope or regression coefficient (m) and intercept (c) are

$$m = \frac{\Sigma xy}{\Sigma x^2}$$

this is derived from

$$\Sigma x^2 = \Sigma X_i^2 - \frac{(\Sigma X_i)^2}{n}$$

$$\Sigma xy = \Sigma X_i . Y_i - \frac{\Sigma X_i . \Sigma Y_i}{n}$$

$$c = \bar{Y} - m\bar{X}$$

The degree of correlation between two sets of data can be assessed by calculating the correlation coefficient (r). This will vary between +1 and −1. The proportion of the variation in the value of Y which is the result of the variation in X is given by the value of r^2. This is also known as the proportion of the explained variation. The complement $(1 - r^2)$ is the proportion of unexplained variation. Evaluating whether or not a particular correlation coefficient would have occurred by chance alone involves the calculation of the 't' statistic. This is then inspected in the appropriate 't' table under (n − 2) degrees of freedom, where n is the number of pairs of data. If this shows that there is no correlation this means that the only valid line to draw through the data is one which is parallel with the x axis.

$$r = \frac{\Sigma xy}{\sqrt{\Sigma x^2 . \Sigma y^2}}$$

Where Σxy and Σx^2 are derived as above and

$$\Sigma y^2 = \Sigma Y_i^2 - \frac{(\Sigma Y_i)^2}{n}$$

From this

$$t = \sqrt{\frac{r^2(n-2)}{1-r^2}}$$

For a fuller explanation of the uses and limits of statistical methods the reader is referred to:

Siegel S S 1956 Non-parametric statistics for the behavioural sciences. McGraw-Hill, Kogakusha, Tokyo
Snedecor G W, Cochran W G 1967 Statistical methods, 6th edn. Iowa State University, Ames, Iowa
Bernstein L, Wetherall M 1952 Statistics for medical and other biological students. Livingstone, Edinburgh
Croxton F E 1959 Elementary statistics with applications in medicine and the biological sciences. Dover, New York

Index

Accuracy, 3
  average level, 4
  blood group serology, in 34–35
  changes in, 153–158
    control charts, 154
    Cusum charts, 154–158
    control schemes, in 166–167
Anticoagulants, 52, 54, 56
  blood/anticoagulant ratio, 52
  citrate *see* Citrate
  control of, 52, 56–57
    British system, 56–57
  heparin *see* Heparin
  National Reference Laboratory for Anticoagulant Reagents and Control (NRLARC), 52
  see also Clotting factors, Prothrombin time, Thromboplastin reagents
Antiglobin testing, 38, 41–49
  antiglobin reagent, 44
  cell concentration, 42
  cell volume, 42–43
  cell washes, 43–44
  centrifugation, 44–45
  direct, 49
  error rates, 38, 41–42
  external proficiency testing, 38, 41–49
  incubation time, 43
  indirect, 48–49
  recommended techniques, 48–49
  result reading, 45
  serum volume, 42–43
  standardisation, 46–49
  tube size, 44
  UK National External Quality Assessment Scheme, 41–49
  wash volume, 44
Antithrombin III (At III), 74–75
  assay, 74–75
  deficiency, 74
  heparin assay, 75
  international reference preparation, 75
Automated instruments,
  batch assays, 98–99
  cell counting, 19–20
    calibration, 30
    maintenance, 19–20
    platelets, 27

Automated instruments (*cont'd*)
    red cells, 23
    white cells, 21
  control samples, 160–169
  Coulter counter *see* Coulter counter
  hematocrit, 25
  hemoglobin, 16–17
  red cell indices, 26

Batch assays, 87–101
  control materials, 99–100
  error, 91
    laboratory components, 91
    physiological components, 91
  instrumentation, 97–99
    automated, 98–99
    log books, 95–96
    non-automated, 98
    performance tests for, 99
  interlaboratory control, 93–95
    reference ranges, 94–95
  methods, 91
    accuracy assessment, 92–93
    correction, 96
    evaluation, 91–92, 95
    reproducibility, 92
  proficiency testing programs, 93
  reagents, 97
  standard operating procedure (SOP) *see* Standard operating procedure
Binomial distribution *see* Distribution
Blood counting, 13–33, 103–120
  automated *see* Automated instruments
  cell size distribution, 31
  coefficient of variation, 19
  hemoglobin *see* Hemoglobin
  interlaboratory trials *see* Interlaboratory trials
  manual, 19
  PCV *see* Packed cell volume
  preparation of control material, 115–120
  primary standard *see* Cyanmethemoglobin
  red cell indices *see* Red cell indices
  red cells *see* Red cell counting
  secondary standards *see* Blood standards
  white cells *see* White cell counting
Blood group serology, external proficiency testing, 34–50
  antibody detection and identification, 38–40

Blood group serology (cont'd)
  antiglobin test *see* Antiglobin testing
  Centre for Disease Control (CDC) 36, 39, 40–41
  College of American Pathologists (CAP) *see* College of American Pathologists
  compatibility testing 40–41
  complicated ABO and Rh(D) grouping 37–38
  error rates *see* Error rates
  Ontario Medical Association (OMA) 35–41
  uncomplicated ABO and Rh(D) grouping, 35–37
  UK National Quality Assessment Scheme, 41–49
Blood standards,
  autoanalyser, 121–122, 161–163
  clotting assays, 67–68
  Coulter 4C *see* Coulter counter
  Factor VIII *see* Factor VIII
  Factor IX *see* Factor IX
  fixed platelets, 119–120
  fresh whole blood, 16–17, 103
  hemolysate, 115–116
  hemoglobin *see* Hemoglobin
  platelets, 29
  primary *see* Cyanmethemoglobin
  prothrombin time, 57–59
  'pseudo-white' cells, 117–118
  secondary, 13
  stability, 122–123
British Comparative Thromboplastin (BCT) *see* Thromboplastin reagents
British Corrected Ratio (BCR) *see* Thromboplastin reagents
Bureau of Biologics (BoB)
  Factor VIII standard, 70

Cell size distribution, 31–32
Citrate,
  anticoagulant, 52–53, 54
Clotting factors, 54, 67–76
  antithrombin III (At III) *see* Antithrombin III
  assays *see* Coagulation assays
  biosynthesis, 54
  Factor II, 73
  Factor VII, 73
  Factor VIII *see* Factor VIII
  Factor X, 73
  Factor IX *see* Factor IX
  fibrinogen *see* Fibrinogen
  heparin *see* Heparin
  oral anticoagulants, 54
  percentage in reference plasma, 58
  prothrombin time, effect on 54
  stability in reference plasma, 58
  thrombin, 74
  vitamin K, 54
Coagulation assays, 51–52, 67–77
  antithrombin III *see* Antithrombin III
  control samples, 68–69
  Factor VIII *see* Factor VIII
  Factor IX *see* Factor IX

Coagulation (cont'd)
  fibrinogen *see* Fibrinogen
  heparin *see* Heparin
  standards, 67–69
    normal plasma, 67
    stable reference, 67–68
  thrombin, 74
  see also Coagulation tests
Coagulation tests, 51–67
  blood collection, 52
  National Institute for Biological Standards and Control (NIBSC)
  National Reference Laboratory for Anticoagulant Reagents and Control (NRLARC)
  partial thromboplastin time *see* Partial thromboplastin time
  prothrombin time *see* Prothrombin time
  see also Coagulation assays
Cold agglutinates, 17
  mean cell volume, and, 25
College of American Pathologists (CAP), surveys
  blood counting, 102
  blood group serology, 35–41
  fibrinogen assay, 74
  prothrombin time, 59–60
Compatibility testing, 40–41
  UK National External Quality Assessment Scheme, 41–49
Control charts, 2, 8, 9
  control samples, use with, 154, 159
  disadvantages, 154
  historical development, 2
  limits, 9
  sensitivity, 158
  Shewhart, 154, 158
Control samples, intralaboratory quality control, 151–172
  accuracy, 166–167
  analysing results, 153–154, 165–166
  calculations, 169–170
  control charts *see* Control charts
  control preparation, 152
  corrective action, 166
  cusum charts *see* Cusum charts
  frequency of analysis, 153, 164
  precision monitoring, 166–169
  stability, 170
  standard preparation, 152
  test procedure, 160
  variation, 170–171
  see also Whole blood control
Coulter counter,
  Coulter 4C, 17, 174
    cyanmethemoglobin conversion time, 17–18
    lysis, 17
    red cell indices, 174
  optical system, 17–19
  patterns of change in red cell indices, 137–143
  whole blood control, 151–152
  see also Automated instruments

INDEX

Cumulative sum (Cusum) procedures, 8–12
  advantages, 10
  application, 11
  chart construction, 10–11
  control results, for, 154–157, 159–160
  decision rule, 11
  mask construction, 11
  sensitivity, 158
  target value (T), 10
Cyanmethemoglobin (ICSH hemoglobincyanide) 13
  Beer's Law and, 14
  conversion time from hemoglobin, 15, 17–19
    Coulter 4C, 17
    fresh blood, 17
  photometer calibration, 14
  primary standard, 13
  stability, 15

Differential leukocyte count, 177–178
  accuracy, 177
    neutrophils, 177
  cell number, 177
  coefficient of variation, 177
Direct antiglobin test *see* Antiglobin testing
Distribution, 6
  Binomial, 6
  Normal (Gaussian), 7, 112
  Poisson, 6
    change in, 8
Drabkin's reagent, for hemoglobin measurement, 13
  alternative reagents, 14–15
  hemoglobin assay *see* Hemoglobin
  stability, 16

Environmental Protection Agency (EPA) 89
Error rates, 35–47
  ABO and Rh(D) grouping, 35–38
  antibody detection and identification, 38–40
  antiglobin test, 38, 42–47
  compatibility testing, 40–41
External Quality Assessment (EQA) 102

Factor VIII, 70–73
  freeze dried concentrate, 70–71
  international standard (IS) 70, 71
  normal plasma range, 70
  one stage assay, 71, 72
  plasma standard, 70, 71–72
  proficiency assessment, 72–73
  reagents, 72
  techniques, 72
  two stage assay, 71, 72, 81
Factor IX, 73
Fibrinogen assay, 73–74
Food and Drug Administration (FDA) 89

Good laboratory practice (GLP) 89

Hematocrit *see* Packed cell volume

Hemocytometry *see* Platelet counting
Hemoglobin, 13–19
  automation *see* Automated instruments
  calibration verification, 145, 146
  conversion time to cyanmethemoglobin *see* Cyanmethemoglobin
  interlaboratory trial, 104–107
  method, 13–19
  reagent *see* Drabkin's reagent
  red cell indices, and, 123–124
  standards, 14, 15, 16, 17
    cyanmethemoglobin *see* Cyanmethemoglobin
    commercial, 15
    variation, 174, 176
Hemophilia therapy, 70
  Factor VIII assay, 70
Heparin assay, 75–77
  antithrombin III interaction *see* Antithrombin III
  anti-Xa, 75–77
  standard curve, 76
  variability, 75–77

ICSH hemoglobincyanide *see* Cyanmethemoglobin
Indirect antiglobin test *see* Antiglobin testing
Interlaboratory trials, in routine blood counting, 102–120
  analysis of results, 104–107
  batch assays *see* Batch assays
  blood group serology *see* Blood group serology
  coagulation tests, 51–52
  control material, 103, 115–120
    see also Blood standards
  poor performance, 105–106, 112–114
    clinical significance, 113–114
    recognition, 112–114
    statistical analysis, 112–113
    target values, 114
International quality control, 102
Intralaboratory control, 120–172
  control samples, using *see* Control samples
  patient data, using *see* Red cell indices

Laboratory results, interpretation and significance, 173–181
  methodological constancy, 173–176
    control materials, 173
    difficulties, 173
    red cell indices, 173–175
  morphological studies *see* Morphology
  physiological variation, 176–178
    physiological variation (cont)
      differential leukocyte count, 177
      hemoglobin, 176
      platelets, 177
      red cell count, 176
      red cell indices, 176
Latex particles *see* Cell size distribution
Lyse S
  hemoglobin concentration, and 17

INDEX

Mean cell hemoglobin (MCH) 26
　see also Red cell indices
Mean cell hemoglobin concentration (MCHC) 26
　see also Red cell indices
Mean cell volume (MCV) 25–26
　automated hematocrit calculation, 26
　electrical impedence method, 25
　microhematocrit method, 25
　sources of error, 25–26
　stability, 123–125
　trapped plasma correction, 128
　see also Red cell indices
Manchester Comparative Reagent (MCR) see Prothrombin time
Morphology, 178–181
　bone marrow smears, 180
　interpretation, 180–181
　Laboratory Proficiency Testing Program (LPTP) 178–180

National Institute for Biological Standards and Control (NIBSC) 70
　British working standard for Factor VIII, 70
Neutrophil count see Differential leukocyte count
Normal (Gaussian) distribution see Distribution

Oral anticoagulants see Anticoagulants

Packed cell volume (PCV) 25–26
　electrical impedance method, 25
　MCV calculation see Mean cell volume
　microhematocrit method, 25
　　EDTA, effect of 25
　　plasma trapping, effect of 25
Partial thromboplastin time (PTT) 63–67
　activated (APTT) 63–67
　　activation time, 64–65
　　activator, 64–65
　　heparin, effect of 64–65
　　method, 78–79
　　phospholipid see Phospholipid
　　technical variables, 63
　non-activated (NAPTT) 63
　standardization, 66–67
　　clotting factor deficiency, 66
　　heparin therapy, 66–67
　　standard cephalin extract, 66
　　US survey, 66
Patient data, use in intralaboratory quality control see Red cell indices
Phospholipid, for partial thromboplastin time, 65
　activation time, 64
　activity, 65
　cephalin, 63, 66, 78–79
　diluent, 64
　Factor VIII deficiency, 66
　oxidation, 65
　preparation, 80
PIVKA proteins,
　artificially produced plasma, in 58
　formation of, 54
　prothrombin activity, and 55

Platelets, 26–30, 119–120
　counting see Platelet counting
　fixed, 119–120
Platelet counting, 26–30
　background counts, 29
　electronic, 27–30
　　calibration, 28–29
　　diluted whole blood, 27–28
　　platelet rich plasma, 27–28
　　sample dilution, 29–30
　　size distribution, 30
　hemocytometry, 26–27
　　coefficient of variation, 27
　　reference method, 27
　physiological variation, 177
　reference materials, 29
　specimen quality, 29
Poisson distribution see Distribution
Precision, 3
　changes in, 158–160
　　control charts, 159
　　Cusum charts, 159–160
　control scheme, in 166–167
　dispersion, 4
　　range, 4
　　standard deviation, 5
　　variance, 5
Prothrombin activity see Prothrombin time
Prothrombin index see Prothrombin time
Prothrombin ratio see Prothrombin time
Prothrombin time, 53–62, 77–78
　benchmark system, 59–60
　clotting factors see Clotting factors
　clotting time, 55
　international standardization, 60–62
　method, 77–78
　oral anticoagulants, effect of, see Anticoagulants
　PIVKA proteins see PIVKA proteins
　proficiency assessment scheme, 57
　ratio, 54–55, 77
　reference plasma, 57–59
　　stability, 58
　　variation, 58
　results, 55
　　prothrombin activity, 55
　　prothrombin index, 55
　　prothrombin ratio, 55
　technical variables, 54–56
　see also Thromboplastin reagents
Pulse generators, cell counter calibration, 30–31

Red blood cells,
　counting see Red cell counting
　fixed, 116–117
　indices see Red cell indices
Red cell counting, 23–25
　adherence to counting vial, 24
　cell size distribution, 31
　cell volume, 23–24
　coefficient of variation, 176
　detergent, 23–24

INDEX 191

Red cell counting (*cont'd*)
  instrument calibration, 23
  lytic agents, 24–25
  plasticisers, 24–25
  Coulter 4C, in, 174
  diagnosis of disease, use in, 123
  instrument calibration, 127, 136
  intra-laboratory quality control using patient data, 123–150
    off line implementation, 129–130
    on line implementation, 130
    patterns of change in data plots *see* Coulter counter
  MCH *see* Mean cell hemoglobin
  MCHC *see* Mean cell hemoglobin concentration
  MCV *see* Mean cell volume
  mean, 125–127
    averaging algorithm, 126–127
    comparison of, 127, 128
    estimation of, 125–127
    sample size, 125–126
  stability, 123–124
  variation, 173–175
    study results, 174–175

Shewart control chart *see* Control charts
Standard operating procedure (SOP) 89–91
Statistics, 1–12, 182–185
  accuracy *see* Accuracy
  coefficient of variation, 183
  control charts *see* Control charts
  Cusum procedures *see* Cumulative sum procedures
  distribution *see* Distribution
  location *see* Accuracy
  mean, 4–5, 182
  population, 5
  precision *see* Precision
  probability, 6
  sample, 5
    size, 10, 183
  standard deviation, 5, 182–183
  standard error, 5
  stochastic models, 8–9
  students t test, 183–184
  variance, 5, 182–184
Stochastic models *see* Statistics

Target value *see* Cusum procedires
Thrombin *see* Clotting factors

Thromboplastin reagents,
  British Comparative Thromboplastin (BCT) 57
  British Corrected Ratio (BCR) 56
  Manchester Comparative Reagent (MCR) 56
  prothrombin time ratio, 54–55, 57
  quantitative comparison of, 79
  reference, 60
    international, 62
  variation, 54–55
  see also Anticoagulants, Prothrombin time
Thromboplastin time, partial *see* Partial prothrombin time
t test *see* Statistics

United Kingdom External Quality Assessment Scheme,
  blood group serology, 41–49
  hemoglobin trial, 104–107
  routine blood counting, 103

White blood cells, 21–23, 117–118
  counting *see* White cell counting
  pseudo 117–118
White cell counting, 21–23
  background count, 23
  biological variability, 23
  cell size distribution, 21, 31
  coefficient of variation, 176
  differential counts *see* Differential leukocyte count
  dilution, 21
  instrumentation, 21–23
    aperture tube, 21, 22
    calibration, 22–23
    coincidence correction, 21
    pulse height, 21–22
  lytic agent, 21, 22, 23
  sources of error, 21–22
Whole blood control,
  accuracy, 166
  analysis of results, 165–166
  automated blood counter *see* Coulter counter
  frequency of analysis, 164
  handling, 163
  mean and variance, 163–164
  precision, 166–169
  preparation, 161–163
    fixed chicken red cells, 161
    partial fixation of human red cells, 161–162
  quality control limits, 163–164
  see also Control samples